Health Care Reform
in Radiology

T0176799

To the memory of Gunther Semelka and Joseph Armao

Health Care Reform in Radiology

Richard C. Semelka
University of North Carolina at Chapel Hill
Department of Radiology
School of Medicine
North Carolina
USA

and

Jorge Elias Jr
The School of Medicine of Ribeirao Preto
University of Sao Paulo
Sao Paulo
Brazil

WILEY Blackwell

Library of Congress Cataloging-in-Publication Data:
Semelka, Richard C., author.
  Health care reform in radiology / Richard C. Semelka and Jorge Elias Jr.
      p. ; cm.
  Includes bibliographical references and index.
  ISBN 978-1-118-64217-7 (pbk. : alk. paper) – ISBN 978-1-118-64221-4 (ePDF) –
ISBN 978-1-118-64227-6 – ISBN 978-1-118-64229-0 (ePub) – ISBN 978-1-118-64236-8 (eMobi)
  I. Elias, Jorge, Jr, author. II. Title.
  [DNLM: 1. Radiology–economics–United States.   2. Radiology–trends–United States.
3. Costs and Cost Analysis–United States.   4. Health Care Reform–United States.   5. Quality of
Health Care–United States.   6. Unnecessary Procedures–economics–United States. WN 100]
  RC78.15
  616.07'570681–dc23
                            2013018319

Printed in Singapore

10 9 8 7 6 5 4 3 2 1

Contents

Color plate section can be found facing page 184

Contributors

Diane Armao
University of North Carolina at Chapel Hill, School of Medicine, Department of Radiology and Pathology and Laboratory Medicine, Chapel Hill, North Carolina, USA

Michael Brand
Department of Radiology, University Hospital of Erlangen, Erlangen, Germany

Lauren M. B. Burke
University of North Carolina at Chapel Hill, School of Medicine, Department of Radiology, Chapel Hill, North Carolina, USA

Jorge Elias Jr
The School of Medicine of Ribeirao Preto, University of Sao Paulo, Brazil

Michael A. Kuefner
Department of Radiology, University Hospital of Erlangen, Erlangen, Germany

Richard C. Semelka
University of North Carolina at Chapel Hill, School of Medicine, Department of Radiology, Chapel Hill, North Carolina, USA

John Stonestreet
Hopecare Clinical Solutions, Chapel Hill, North Carolina, USA

Michael Uder
Department of Radiology, University Hospital of Erlangen, Erlangen, Germany

Preface

"Patients first" was the motto for the 98th Assembly and Meeting of the Radiological Society of North America (RSNA). Our intention of writing this book is to provide a road map to achieve that goal. We describe major issues in health care that affect Radiology and describe for each of these ideal and workable solutions. The subjects we cover in this book encompass some novel concepts that we believe will be valuable additions to the practice of Radiology. Foremost among these are: recommendations for development and adoption of what we have termed Diagnostic Imaging Appropriateness Score, as a measure to determine if a study should be performed; anonymous evaluation of radiologist's performance; holding medical experts legally accountable for their opinions if they differ from the norm; incorporation of radiologists serving as blinded reviewers in medicolegal cases as a method to obtain continuing education credits; and that the US health care system should emulate the Australian system as a model. We believe that the recommendations we have provided would serve to dramatically improve the quality and safety of Radiology practice. As with most important improvements, there has to be the will to change before it is too late, and these improvements will certainly need the involvement of the entire Radiology community as well as governmental agencies.

Richard C. Semelka
Jorge Elias Jr

CHAPTER 1

Health care reform: The scope of the problem

Richard C. Semelka,[1] Diane Armao,[2] and Jorge Elias Jr[3]

[1] University of North Carolina at Chapel Hill, School of Medicine, Department of Radiology, Chapel Hill, NC, USA
[2] University of North Carolina at Chapel Hill, School of Medicine, Department of Radiology and Pathology and Laboratory Medicine, Chapel Hill, NC, USA
[3] The School of Medicine of Ribeirao Preto, University of Sao Paulo, Brazil

There is virtually no disagreement that serious problems exist in the US health care system. Prodigal outlays for medical care are undeniable. From a global perspective, the USA pays more per capita in health care than any other country and yet ranks 37th in the world regarding quality of health care; in part this is because approximately 45 million individuals (1 in 6.5) remain uninsured. From a national perspective, per capita Medicare spending in different parts of the country varies dramatically. Medicare enrollees in higher spending regions receive more care than those in lower spending regions but do not have increased access to care, better quality care, improved health outcomes or patient satisfaction [1]. Moreover, there even exists a negative association between higher health care expenditures and outcomes, such as mortality at the regional level [2]. The notion that additional growth in health care cost is primarily driven by advances in science and technology and that more spending will result in improved quality of care is no longer tenable.

Radiologists are ideally positioned to discuss health care issues from a physician's perspective. Due to the nature of their specialty, radiologists are the main diagnostic consultants for virtually all branches of medical practice and hence are familiar with the breadth of medical care. Based on the range of their experience, radiologists can help guide the mechanics involved in health care costs, patient safety and comparative effectiveness metrics. Costs and appropriateness criteria relate to evaluating whether

Health Care Reform in Radiology, First Edition. Richard C. Semelka and Jorge Elias Jr.
© 2013 John Wiley & Sons, Inc. Published 2013 by John Wiley & Sons, Inc.

certain diagnostic studies are warranted, while patient safety addresses issues centered on radiation dose reduction in imaging studies, including substitution of alternate examinations in particular clinical settings. In order to achieve these goals, accurate patient information is paramount.

The waste and the cost

As pointed out by the US Congressional Research Service in 2007 the USA spends more money on health care than any other country in the Organisation for Economic Co-operation and Development (OECD), which comprises 30 countries that represent the most economically advanced countries in the world. The USA spent $6102 per capita on health care in 2004; double that spent by OECD and 19.9% more than Luxembourg, the second-highest spending country. In that year, 15.3% of the US economy was devoted to health care, compared with 8.9% in the average OECD country and 11.6% in second-placed Switzerland. The OECD has stated that US prices for medical care commodities and services are significantly higher than in other countries and serve as a key determinant of higher overall spending.

One striking example of high health care costs has been recently reported in McAllen, Texas, which possesses the lowest US household income but has the second most expensive US health care market, spending twice the national average [3, 4]. Indeed, patients in McAllen get more diagnostic testing, more hospital treatment, more surgery, and more home care compared to any another town, with no recognition of overall quantity by hospital administrators [3, 4].

In a 2008 analysis by Price Waterhouse Health Research Institute (PwC) on sources of financial waste in the US health care system, there was approximately $1 trillion in waste, comprising more than a half the total spending, with $200 billion attributable to defensive health care practice [5]. However, due to the ubiquitous nature of defensive health care practice, such cost may be considerably underestimated.

The PwC indicates that the recession that began in 2007 has changed the trend of medical cost in the USA. Medical cost had a surprisingly low growth rate of 7.5% in 2010, after an estimate of 9%, but increased to 8% in 2011 and was expected to increase to 8.5% in 2012. This trend represents the projected increase in the costs of medical services assumed in setting premiums for health insurance plans. The largest single component of spending is physician services, which accounts for about 33%

of all benefit costs. Outpatient hospital services and prescriptions account for 17% and 15%, respectively. Other services such as home health, skilled nursing, and medical equipment account for a meager 4% of benefit costs.

Expectations surrounding US government health reform, as manifested by the American Reinvestment and Recovery Act of 2009 and the Patient Protection and Affordable Care Act of 2010 (PPACA), will certainly contribute to cost shifting, but the magnitude of its impact on cost-ineffective services versus more cost-effective but underutilized services is not completely clear. One likely scenario involves physicians and hospitals being paid higher levels of compensation for more cost-effective services relative to their costs but lower levels of payment at or below cost for less cost-effective services [6]. Actually, the American College of Radiology recently dedicated a whole issue of the *Journal of the American College of Radiology* (JACR) to this issue, bringing various aspects related to cost, utilization, value and coverage regarding the US Health Reform [7–14]. What seems more than certain is that US health care reform, one way or another, will dominate the scenario of change for patients, physicians, and all other stakeholders for years to come—all hope for a change to the better.

The causes: Expanded list

Because of the intrinsic complexity of the problem and the multifactorial nature of causality, it is not an easy task to determine the main causes of high medical costs, since they can change over time due to multiple confounding factors. A dominant influence is also the subjective bias of the interested observer's point of view. Interestingly, this can also explain why many have failed to present a definitive solution, and few have attempted to address the core of the problem.

Nonetheless, certain causes are clearly identifiable as reflecting a "frequent flyer" list irrespective of the observer's role in the US health care system, or self-interest as a stakeholder.

An attempt to categorize these causes was made by PwC, and they grouped them as follows: 1) behavioral—where individual behaviors are shown to lead to health problems, and have compromised opportunities for earlier, preventative interventions; 2) operational—where administrative or other business processes appear to add costs without creating value; and 3) clinical—where medical care itself is considered inappropriate, entailing overuse, misuse or under-use of particular interventions, missed

---

Box 1.1 Basic list of rising medical costs in the USA

Physician shortages and high prices of physicians' services
Medical litigation
Defensive medicine
Excessive ordering of expensive medical tests
Excessive charge per procedure
Spending on pharmaceuticals
Small or no success to address preventable health risk factors (such as obesity,
    smoking, and alcohol abuse)
Excessive health care expenditure on the terminally ill
Health care fraud

---

opportunities for earlier interventions, and overt errors leading to poor quality care for the patient and added health care cost.

A basic but yet expanded list of rising medical costs is presented in Box 1.1. These causes will be discussed in more detail in this publication.

References

1. Fisher ES, Wennberg DE, Stukel TA, Gottlieb DJ, Lucas FL, Pinder EL. The implications of regional variations in Medicare spending. Part 1: The content, quality, and accessibility of care. Ann Intern Med 2003; 138:273–287.
2. Fisher ES, Wennberg DE, Stukel TA, Gottlieb DJ, Lucas FL, Pinder EL. The implications of regional variations in Medicare spending. Part 2: Health outcomes and satisfaction with care. Ann Intern Med 2003; 138:288–298.
3. Gawande AA, Fisher ES, Gruber J, Rosenthal MB. The cost of health care—highlights from a discussion about economics and reform. N Engl J Med 2009; 361:1421–1423.
4. Kauffman-Pickelle C. Radiology and the Culture of Money. ImagingBiz 2009. Available online at: http://www.imagingbiz.com/articles/view/radiology-and-the-culture-of-money1 [accessed February 19, 2013].
5. The price of excess: Identifying waste in healthcare spending. Report Document from PricewaterhouseCoopers' Health Research Institute 2008; 22. Available online at: http://www.pwc.com/us/en/healthcare/publications/the-price-of-excess.jhtml [accessed February 19, 2013].
6. Weinstein MC, Skinner JA. Comparative effectiveness and health care spending—implications for reform. N Engl J Med 2010; 362:460–465.
7. Rawson JV. Roots of health care reform. J Am Coll Radiol 2012; 9:684–688.
8. Norbash A, Hindson D, Heineke J. The accountable health care act of Massachusetts: Mixed results for an experiment in universal health care coverage. J Am Coll Radiol 2012; 9:734–739.

9. Lexa FJ. A radiologist's guide to the federal election of 2012: What you should know before you go into the booth. J Am Coll Radiol 2012; 9:740–744.

10. Lexa FJ. Drivers of health reform in the United States: 2012 and beyond. J Am Coll Radiol 2012; 9:689–693.

11. Lee CI, Enzmann DR. Measuring radiology's value in time saved. J Am Coll Radiol 2012; 9:713–717.

12. Duszak R, Jr, Berlin JW. Utilization management in radiology, part 1: Rationale, history, and current status. J Am Coll Radiol 2012; 9:694–699.

13. Duszak R, Jr, Berlin JW. Utilization management in radiology, part 2: Perspectives and future directions. J Am Coll Radiol 2012; 9:700–703.

14. Carlos RC, Rawson JV. Introduction to the special issue-health care reform: Darkness before dawn? J Am Coll Radiol 2012; 9:682–683.

CHAPTER 2

Only studies which are necessary

Diane Armao,[1] Jorge Elias Jr,[2] and Richard C. Semelka[3]

[1] University of North Carolina at Chapel Hill, School of Medicine, Department of Radiology and Pathology and Laboratory Medicine, Chapel Hill, NC, USA
[2] The School of Medicine of Ribeirao Preto, University of Sao Paulo, Brazil
[3] University of North Carolina at Chapel Hill, School of Medicine, Department of Radiology, Chapel Hill, NC, USA

Components critical to evaluating whether imaging studies are necessary include: 1) an intermediate to high pre-test probability patient population; 2) the seriousness of the disease entity; 3) the treatability of the disease process (taking into consideration lesion size and stage of disease); 4) the sensitivity, specificity, predictive values, and accuracy of the test; 5) the safety of the procedure, including ionizing radiation and incidence and severity of complications; 6) the nature and number of prior imaging studies for the same clinical condition; and 7) the comparative effectiveness with other approaches, including, importantly, doing no test.

Scope of the issue

Quality health care, according the National Committee for Quality Assurance (NCQA) is defined as "the extent to which patients get the care they need in a manner that most effectively protects or restores their health" [1]. As described by the Patient-Centered Outcomes Research Institute (PCORI), an increasing body of clinical comparative effectiveness research (CCER) compares the relative effectiveness and safety of alternative, preventative, diagnostic, or treatment options [2]. A high priority of CCER is to evaluate the health effects of clinical practices that have

---

been widely adapted by clinicians, despite limited evidence about the risks and benefits [3].

Clinical practice is oftentimes shaped by the dominant and pervasive influence of available diagnostic imaging. In turn, powerful imaging marketing strategies focusing on profit engenders the rapid purchase of machines prior to completely understanding how this technology should be implemented to improve outcomes [4]. Such dynamics between the ease of acceptance in clinical practice and the lure of profitable marketing and investment has created excess imaging capacity, confounded by few evidence-based guidelines for its use. A study published in a premier public health care and policy journal addressed the problem of rapid expansion of diagnostic imaging in the face of limited, measurable health outcomes [5]. To illustrate this issue, using census data on imaging units and Medicare claims data, the authors investigated the rapid diffusion of computed tomography angiography (CTA) use for assessing abdominal–pelvic abnormalities, including abdominal aortic aneurysm, versus catheter angiography. Patients who newly received the less invasive CTA but would not have received catheter angiography before could have benefited if the additional screening depicted disease that would have gone undetected before. To provide some evidence of this, the authors analyzed whether the additional diagnostic testing was associated with changes in therapeutic procedure rates. Such treatment rates provide a key mechanism by which improved health outcomes might be expected to occur. If expanded availability and use of diagnostic imaging catches treatable conditions, and conditions that merit treatment, the authors expected to observe a higher rate of therapeutic procedures, including direct repairs for ruptured aneurysms, endovascular repairs, and endarterectomies [5]. However, the authors concluded that for each additional 100 CTA users in a metropolitan area, statistically there were only about 1.1 more beneficiaries who received one or more of these treatments [5].

The role of diagnostic imaging in patient care is costly. In 2007, Medicare expenditures for imaging services totaled $11.4 billion, representing a material increase from the $8.4 billion spent in 2002 [6]. The direct cost of imaging studies is over $100 billion annually [7]. There is serious concern that expensive imaging tests are ordered and performed without an evidence base to support their appropriateness or health benefit [8]. Further, CCER experts argue that there is almost no evidenciary bar at all to gain Food and Drug Administration approval of imaging technologies [9]. No doubt, technologic and diagnostic capabilities in imaging have soared over recent years due, in part, to an ever enlarging enterprise of research. Yet, research that quantifies the long-term effects of imaging on patient outcomes remains disproportionately sparse [6].

Hence little of what is termed evidence-based medicine is actually evidence-based—mainly because the proxies used for evidence are short term or only examine a portion of the clinical picture, rather than long term and evaluating the totality of the patient's condition. Experience has shown that limited perspective evidence-based studies ultimately are often shown to have little to no merit. We have to train ourselves to look at the whole picture and for longer time periods. In particular, radiologists, as physician and patient providers, need to work to become better informed of the natural history of the diseases we evaluate, as excessive imaging may not only be more expensive but also be worse than the disease itself. Besides the personal health costs of over-radiation, unnecessary advanced diagnostic imaging has engendered an epidemic of indeterminate, incidental findings at least as troubling to both physician and patient as the events that prompted the initial imaging exam [10]. The author of a recent editorial in *Imaging for the Clinician Special Section* laments "I know radiologists who have never seen a normal CT exam. They dictate 2-page reports describing in excruciating detail every dot in the lung bases, liver, spleen and kidney; every top normal lymph node is measured, every benign ovarian cyst is described, every hedge is sat upon. To make matters worse, each of these heroic poems ends with recommendations for further imaging to include ultrasound (US) of the pelvis, US of the kidneys, magnetic resonance imaging of the pelvis, CT of the full chest, and repeat studies with additional contrast or thin-section evaluations of specific organs for the 'ditzels' described. What is a well-meaning clinician to do with such generally worthless information?" [10].

There is widespread agreement that a considerable number of imaging procedures performed are unnecessary [11–15]. In one publication it was estimated that one-third of CTs are unnecessary [16]. Unfortunately, the current circumstance is aptly comparable to Mark Twain's observation: "many people talk about the weather, but nobody is doing anything about it." Many authorities discuss the problem [17], but concrete proposals are lacking. Hence we have created a heightened environment of anxiety, but with no solutions in sight.

Some publications suggest that 20–50% of high-tech imaging, such as multisection CT, magnetic resonance imaging (MRI), and positron emission tomography (PET), fail to provide information that improves patients' welfare and hence may represent unnecessary imaging services [18]. By definition, *overutilization* may be defined as application of imaging procedures in clinical situations where imaging tests are unlikely to improve patient outcomes [18]. Inappropriate imaging augments health care costs without increasing the quality of health care. Recent research shows that approximately one-third of health care spending is duplicative, unhelpful, or makes patients worse [19]. Unnecessary imaging studies seldom reveal the cause of the patient's complaint yet may reveal incidental findings that require further imaging or interventional procedures to clarify [20]. These further investigations, the so-called "snowball effect," often result in undue anxiety, further imaging, and further therapy that cause more harm than good.

The rapid rise of medical imaging reflects ongoing advances in technology and expanded applications in high-tech modalities. This growth rate is abetted by reflexive acceptance of imaging as standard of care, without an evidence base to create formal practice guidelines. Major causes of inappropriate utilization of medical imaging include: 1) medical liability fears, 2) patient demand, 3) economically motivated in-office self-referral, and 4) physician inexperience and lack of support in the appropriate clinical application of diagnostic imaging [21, 22].

Such a lack of rigorous, systematic compliance with appropriateness criteria has created a serious gap between health care delivery and high-quality patient-centered outcomes. As a case in point, a recent retrospective analysis from an academic medical center of a large group of CT and MRI examinations for appropriateness using evidence-based guidelines revealed that 26% did not meet appropriateness criteria [21]. In this analysis, in the appropriate study group 58% had positive findings that affected medical management, whereas within the inappropriate group only 13% had positive findings that affected management. Notably, the highest percentage of inappropriate examinations was CT studies of the brain without contrast [21]. Additionally, there was a high negativity rate among these inappropriate examinations; the odds were 3.5 times higher that a negative finding would be associated with an inappropriate versus an appropriate examination. This is critical information for policy makers in the pursuit of utilization guidelines for medical imaging. Patients, physicians, payers, and the public should become better informed about the positive predictive value of imaging tests, while simultaneously making the commitment to decrease costs and ensure quality and safety in our nation's health.

In general, imaging appropriateness criteria consist of radiology expert consensus, including the American College of Radiology (ACR) Appropriateness Criteria and the Royal College of Radiology (RCR) Guidelines [23].

Medical imaging appropriateness criteria are often supplemented by indication and procedure pairs created by expert consensus panels of primary care physicians and clinicians in relevant clinical specialties [24]. However, knowledge of imaging appropriateness criteria is not widespread, and utilization is voluntary, resulting in fragmented adherence. Well-designed computerized radiology order entry and decision support systems are particularly well suited to help clinicians navigate through evidence-based guidelines at the point of care [24]. The goals of guidelines such as those of the ACR are important and laudable efforts. A potential problem that has not been evaluated is the actual level of expertise of expert panels, and individuals have a tendency to believe whatever methodology they primarily use is the appropriate one. A further problem with imaging society appropriateness criteria is that although their criteria recommends the best test for a condition (e.g. noncontrast head CT for potential intracranial bleed) they generally provide no guidance whether any study should be performed to begin with. This forms the foundation of the criteria that we propose below that should take both imaging appropriateness and clinical appropriateness into consideration.

Ideal solution

One perfect test for any and all diseases is beyond any achievement in our era. Diseases and microorganisms evolve, and the host component changes, reflecting changes in an aging population, interaction between human and environment, and increasing population size. Probably, the closest to an ideal solution for such complicated problems may be based on a futuristic science-based strategy. Already steps are made toward using genetic information to determine the probability of disease occurrence. The best-known example of this is BRAC1 and BRAC2 for breast cancer. It is not farfetched to imagine that we will be able to detect all possible disease, by searching predisposition through understanding our DNA codes before we are even born and probabilistically determining disease likelihood based on our entire genetic makeup. We anticipate that in that future imaging will maintain an important role in detecting actual disease in individuals who are determined to be at risk, or susceptible, to that particular disease. Imaging will likely not be supplanted, but augmented, by genetic profiling.

In January 2012 the X PRIZE Foundation and Qualcomm Foundation announced the launch of the $10 million Qualcomm Tricorder X PRIZE, a global competition that they claim will revolutionize health care (see http://www.qualcommtricorderxprize.org) [25]. In this competition, teams will leverage technology innovation in areas such as artificial intelligence and wireless sensing—much like the fictional medical Tricorder—to make medical diagnoses independent of a physician or health care provider [25]. A tricorder is a device used by the Star Trek character Dr. Leonard McCoy, a.k.a. "Bones," which he would wave over the body of a subject and instantly discover whatever disease they had, without even touching the individual. Could this be the future?

It is clearly important to have timely and accurate diagnoses of diseases that are treatable, and in many clinical circumstances these diagnoses would be of "pre-malignant" conditions, which ultimately can be cured, prior to the disease becoming frankly malignant. In many of these clinical circumstances diagnosing a disease early may not change the natural history of disease, and controversy exists on this subject for many diseases, including prostate cancer. This is termed lead-time bias, and both the detection of prostate cancer and of breast cancer has been scrutinized with the recognition of this bias in mind. It is our opinion however, and we may be in the majority, that it is always important to recognize disease early. It is appropriate treatment that needs to mature. Worse still, all medical involvement that follows an initial diagnosis, that is more imaging and more treatment, may cause more harm than good, while at the same time be associated with high cost. Some of the most disturbing health care scenarios are the high-cost, highly toxic strategies of some chemotherapy regimens, which may translate into 2 weeks extra of life, rendered miserable because of side effects of the therapy anyway, for $500,000 in added cost. That is why solid medical research is the main foundation to pave the path to a more ideal solution.

Practical solution

Our practical solution was inspired, in part, by the recent Institute of Medicine's (IOM) response to the request of the largest grassroots network of breast cancer survivors and activists in the USA, Susan G. Koman for the Cure, to perform a comprehensive and evidence-based review of environmental causes and risk factors for breast cancer, with a focus on identifying evidence-based actions that can be taken to reduce risk [4, 26]. The IOM concluded that the two environmental factors most strongly associated with breast cancer were combined postmenopausal hormone therapy and exposure to ionizing radiation [26]. Surprising in the IOM review is the emphasis on the *avoidance* of medical imaging as one of the most important steps toward reducing cancer risk [4].

As previously discussed, imaging technology is at the center of the overutilization that has permeated routine practice, oftentimes for medical problems for which there is no evidence of the test's effectiveness or cost-effectiveness; this effect has been termed "test ordering leakage" [27]. We herein propose a platform whereby service provision and quality improvement could occur through the adaptation of a grading scheme or an "imaging scorecard" to assess *appropriate* versus *avoidable* imaging. The imaging scorecard, which we term the Diagnostic Imaging Appropriateness Score (DIAS), would be used to increase the effectiveness of imaging and close the "performance gap" between inappropriate imaging and health care quality improvement. Our development of DIAS takes into consideration both the appropriateness of the imaging test in general (analogous to the ACR appropriateness criteria) but also the appropriateness of imaging specifically for the suspected clinical indications, which at present remains unaddressed. We recommend a scoring system like the Glasgow Coma scale, as scoring systems of this type are already accepted and in use in medical practice, and therefore are readily relatable to practicing physicians.

The fields used to evaluate whether studies are likely to be appropriate or avoidable include all of the following.

1. Pretest probability (PTP), based on patient history, risk factors, and physical examination. PTP classified as: 1 minimal (<5%), 2 low (<15%), 3 intermediate (15–40%), and 4 high (>40%).
2. Seriousness of the disease entity, classified as: 1 not serious, 2 mildly serious, 3 moderately serious (quite debilitating but generally not lethal), and 4 serious (potentially lethal).
3. Treatability of the disease process (taking into consideration lesion size and stage of disease), classified as: 1 not treatable (this can either reflect that the condition is lethal and also the opposite extreme where it is so minor that it is not worth treating), 2 mildly treatable, 3 moderately treatable, and 4 highly treatable.
4. Sensitivity and specificity of the test, classified as: 1 poor, 2 mildly sensitive and specific, 3 moderately sensitive and specific, and 4 very sensitive and specific.
5. Safety of the procedure, including the radiation dose (mSv) and incidence and severity of complications (taking into consideration use of intravenous contrast agents and single study versus multiple study

safety), classified as: 1 very unsafe, 2 mildly safe, 3 moderately safe, and 4 very safe.

6. Presence or absence of repeat imaging studies for the same or other clinical indication. This takes into consideration repeat studies for the same indication and also the type and hence safety of the repeat study. For example, repeat study of the abdomen with noncontrast CT for renal stones, if there have been three studies within the year and all have been negative, maximum points would be deducted for multiple prior studies, the negative results of these studies, and that they were all CT. So multiple studies within the year, all ionizing based and all negative or stable for nonserious disease would confer 1, 2 if this combination suggests that repeat studies have not been excessive or uncalled for, 3 if ionizing radiation studies have been used within the year, and 4 if this is the first ionizing radiation study of the year and there have not been a number (i.e. >2) of nonionizing studies (US or MRI) for similar indications.

7. Comparative effectiveness (CER), emphasizing appropriate imaging tests that could serve as a substitute for CT or other ionizing radiation-based tests (nuclear medicine scintigraphy and PET imaging). The CER that we use here is essentially ACR appropriateness-type criteria, but criteria established by independent observers who are not stakeholders in the procedures themselves. Hence, this means that CER in this context must also take into consideration doing no study whatsoever, for example, similar to the performance of traditional risk factors, laboratory values/Framingham score for the evaluation/prediction of coronary heart disease versus a comparator such as CT coronary artery calcium scores. 1 is poor choice of study, 2 is fair choice of study, 3 is moderately good choice, and 4 is very good choice.

In summary, the system to determine whether an imaging system is indicated includes imaging components and clinical components, analogous to other scales, as used for the Glasgow Coma scale [28] and St. Anne-Mayo grading system for astrocytomas [29]. In total seven components are measured, each rated from 1 to 4, where 1 is minimal indication, 2 is mild indication, 3 is moderate indication, and 4 is strong indication. These values are then added into a composite score, where the total possible value is 28. A lower level should be set below which performing the imaging study is not indicated or marginally indicated, which in the preliminary state we set at 10. This approach differs from other imaging appropriateness systems, which generally evaluate only the imaging components and do not include clinical components. We intend this as a starting point for the assignment of appropriateness to imaging. In our DIAS system the highest score is 28, where we would describe a score of 26–28 as definitely indicated, 22–25 probably indicated, 18–21 possibly indicated (but needs careful clinical scrutiny), 14–17 possibly not indicated, 10–13 probably not indicated, and <10 definitely not indicated.

Our suggestion would also be to use a body of medical experts who do not have a vested interest in these procedures to render an opinion on these determinations, with the obvious requirement that they will solicit input from experts in the field. A logical specialty to render opinions on radiology would be pathologists.

Our scoring scheme is a prototype yet provides a solid workable foundation for future development. For example, as CER is expanded and strengthened in clinical radiology, a criterion for CER is critical. Although we have already included CER in our DIAS system, we recognize that this assessment has not been effectively established. In addition, although still heavily debated as to whether or not economic analysis should be included in CER, we believe that future incorporation of a cost analysis score would be essential in order to evaluate high-value imaging care at a reasonable cost versus expensive low-yield imaging services [6]. Our grading scheme requires tool validation for implementation. Equally important are ongoing multidisciplinary consensus recommendations in order to clearly define clinical scenarios within a patient's entire episode of care, where high-cost imaging can exert the maximum medical benefit.

We will illustrate three common clinical paradigms as examples of how this imaging scorecard DIAS would be implemented.

Example 1: Use of CTA in the evaluation of pulmonary embolism in the emergency department

We have published research that shows that young adults, aged 18–45 years, who undergo pulmonary embolism (PE) CT have a low (5%) incidence of PE [30]. A recent, larger landmark study by Mamlouk et al. revealed that in the setting of no thromboembolic risk factors, it is extraordinarily unlikely (0.95% chance) to have a CT angiogram positive for PE. Another recent large multicenter prospective study, with 11 US emergency departments and 5940 patients enrolled, reported that one-third of imaging performed for suspected PE may be categorized as avoidable [31].

With this as a backdrop, let us look at a CT PE study in a 25-year-old woman with low risk factors, this being the first time study and first CT ever.

1. PTP = 1.
2. Seriousness = 3; taking into consideration that minor distal pulmonary artery emboli are likely best left untreated as the treatment may be worse than the disease.
3. Treatability = 4.
4. Sensitivity = 3; this takes into consideration that although data from the best clinical centers with dedicated teams to optimizing performance and interpretation of these studies is high (95%), in actual clinical practice at the great majority of centers the quality of the study and accuracy of the test approaches 70%.
5. Safety = 1; radiation risk, especially to the breast, is high in this population, but this also considers contrast-induced nephropathy (CIN).
6. CER = 4; contrast-enhanced CT is highly rated as an imaging study using conventional Imaging Society Criteria (ACR appropriateness).
7. Repeated studies = 4; as already mentioned, this was the first CT test performed in this patient.

The DIAS in this patient is 20 of a possible 28 points. Possibly indicated, close clinical evaluation.

Example 2: Use of imaging for low back pain

Low back pain is common. It has a lifetime prevalence of 80% and is the fifth most common reason for all physician visits in the USA [32, 33]. Imaging for low back pain is common, with recent data showing that 42% of patients receive imaging within 1 year [34]. Of these 60% had imaging on the same day as index diagnosis and 80% within 1 month of diagnosis of back pain [34]. Evidence is clear, based on high-quality systematic reviews and meta-analysis, that imaging patients with acute low back pain of less than 6 weeks' duration and no red flag symptoms, defined as severe or progressive neurologic deficits or serious underlying conditions such as cancer or osteomyelitis, results in no clinical benefits [35]. Instead, such avoidable imaging is associated with harms including patient labeling, diminished sense of well-being, radiation exposure, and unnecessary surgery [36].

A recent initiative of the National Physicians Alliance delineated a list of five activities in primary care where changes in practice would foster higher-quality care and ensure more judicious use of finite health care resources [37]. One of the top 5 recommendations was "Do not do imaging for low back pain within the first 6 weeks unless red flags are present" [32, 37].

Although MRI and CT imaging are significantly more costly than standard lumbar radiographs, their use as modalities for spinal imaging in low back pain is increasing [32]. Medicare coverage for MRI of the lumbar spine between 1994 and 2005 increased 307% [38]. Standard lumbar radiographs have such low yield for important common indications, such as disc herniation, that this test is generally of very limited value.

With the above as a backdrop, let us consider a CT of the lumbar spine in a 35-year-old woman within 5 weeks of onset of pain; this is her second CT of the torso within 1 year for various indications:

1. PTP = 1.
2. Seriousness = 2.
3. Treatability = 1; this recognizes that acute onset of back pain in a younger adult is best managed conservatively (also known as: do nothing).
4. Sensitivity = 2; MRI = 4.
5. Safety = 1; medical radiation.
6. CER = 2; MRI is the better study because of superior soft tissue contrast resolution.
7. Repeated studies =2; 1 point deduction for another prior study within the year, and a second point deduction because it was CT (cumulative radiation risk).

Total DIAS score =11. Probably not indicated.

Example 3: Imaging of the liver in a patient with chronic liver disease

A third example is a topic that we have considerable publishing and clinical experience of: imaging of the liver in patients with chronic liver disease [39–46]. In this patient group a primary diagnostic end point is detecting small hepatocellular carcinomas. Let us select a 50-year-old man with Hepatitis C cirrhosis for an annual screening study for hepatocellular carcinoma (HCC). Using contrast-enhanced MRI as the diagnostic test, the following are the evaluations: pt 1 = 4, pt 2 = 4, pt 3 = 4, pt 4 = 4, pt 5 = 4, pt 6 = 4, pt 7 = 4. The DIAS score for MRI is 28, definitely indicated. Substituting in contrast-enhanced CT as the diagnostic test, the evaluations are: pt 1 = 4, pt 2 = 4, pt 3 = 4, pt 4 = 2 (CT is not that sensitive for <2 cm HCCs, which we are targeting with this imaging study), pt 5 = 2 (triple-pass CT is a relatively high radiation exposure, 25 mSv; at 50 years of age he is at mild to moderate risk), pt 6 = 2 (MRI is a better study), pt 7 = 3 (recognizing this is a triple pass we add a 1 point deduction because it is similar to a repeat CT study). The DIAS score for CT in this patient is 21, possibly indicated, clinical assessment. Part of the clinical assessment is that MRI rates 28 and therefore should be used instead. Substituting in noncontrast US, the evaluations are: pt 1 = 4, pt 2 = 4, pt 3 = 4, pt 4 = 1, pt 5 = 4, pt 6 = 2, pt 7 = 4, for a total of 23. This score suggests that US is probably indicated, but the 28 rating of MRI suggests that it is necessary. However, it does also suggest that the use of US is supported in developing countries, where high-quality MRI may not be available. For this patient, the clinical aspects and the safety of the procedure resulted in a higher rating of US over CT, although in most imaging investigations CT may perform slightly better than US for this general disease detection in this patient population from a purely diagnostic standpoint.

An ideal target for DIAS assessment is cardiology imaging practice. Cardiology is unfortunately an especially egregious offender in overutilization of imaging, an illustration of which is that myocardial perfusion imaging (MPI; approximately 9 million studies per year in the USA) is the single test with the highest radiation burden, is often performed multiple times in a given patient, and is considered the "gatekeeper" test for suspected coronary artery disease; this is despite the fact that Patel et al. in the Duke study showed that *only* 38% of patients undergoing invasive coronary angiography had obstructive coronary artery disease [47]. Another recent study reported that multiple testing with MPI was common and in many patients associated with high cumulative estimated doses of radiation [48]. Moreover, more than 80% of initial and 90% of repeat MPI examinations were performed in patients with known cardiac disease or symptoms consistent with it [48].

The presented imaging scorecard used to determine whether a test is necessary or avoidable has two components that are extremely delicate: the seriousness of the disease entity, and the treatability of the disease process (taking into consideration lesion size and stage of disease). Tremendous emotional debate has surrounded this as it applies to excessive health care expenditure on the terminally ill. The famous expression of "death squads" has been used in this context. Approximately 30% of the health care budget is spent on the final 6 months of life [49]. This point clearly has strong ethical and emotional implications as far as denying health care is concerned [50]. Ultimately, to examine the question from a national perspective, it is more beneficial and cost-effective to invest national health care dollars in prevention and early treatment of disease than to pay for a one month's intensive care unit (ICU) stay for a patient with advanced metastatic cancer [13]. The consideration of this point explains why health care costs are so much greater in the USA than in other countries [50]; other countries do not allow terminally ill patients in the ICU, or other extreme health care measures close to the end of life, to this extent, with the benefits realized of only a few extra days of life. The decisions to limit health care have been developed by a number of national health care programs, many of which are based on limiting services using defined age criteria and defined life/wellness functional evaluations [51]. Ultimately, these clinical situations would also be handled when using the formula presented.

Follow-up folly

A second category of overuse is the timing of follow-up studies and the extent to which they are performed. With more than 20 years' clinical experience we have come to realize that we obtain follow-up imaging studies until the patient decides not to come back. This is reminiscent of the dialogue of Woody Allen in the film *Sleeper*, when the principal female character asks Woody the job description of the work he used to do as a stockbroker, and his response is "I invested people's money till it was all gone" [paraphrased]. It is clear that follow-up imaging is excessive, and often serves to over-schedule an important modality that should be a protected resource of health care. Two major drivers of this compulsive behavior are profit and fear of litigation. Although nuances exist for all settings, in general a useful follow-up strategy should not extend beyond 4 years, and the first two follow-ups should be at 3 months (for the possibility of a very serious disease and great imaging uncertainty) or every 6 months (if the disease is less life threatening, or the imaging findings are not so worrisome), with annual follow-up for the next 2 years.

Conclusion

In this chapter we have summarized what we believe to be an important development in health care, which is a quantitative assessment of the likely value of an imaging test. We have also discussed briefly the concept of imaging follow-up.

In chapter 6 we will discuss in more detail the use of systematic, generalizable, evidence-based guidelines embedded within systems such as radiology order entry and decision support.

References

1. National Committee for Quality Assurance. Washington DC. Available online at:http://www.ncqa.org/ [accessed April 23, 2013].
2. PCORI Board of Governors. Developing PCORI's National Priorities for Research and First Research Agenda. In: http://www.pcori.org/assets/Program-Development-Committee-Report.pdf, ed., 2012; 25.
3. Kass N, Faden R, Tunis S. Addressing low-risk comparative effectiveness research in proposed changes to US federal regulations governing research. Jama 2012; 307:1589–1590.
4. Smith-Bindman R. Environmental causes of breast cancer and radiation from medical imaging: findings from the Institute of Medicine report. Arch Intern Med 2012; 172:1023–1027.
5. Baker LC, Atlas SW, Afendulis CC. Expanded use of imaging technology and the challenge of measuring value. Health Aff (Millwood) 2008; 27:1467–1478.
6. Pandharipande PV, Gazelle GS. Comparative effectiveness research: what it means for radiology. Radiology 2009; 253:600–605.
7. Swensen SJ. Patient-centered Imaging. Am J Med 2012; 125:115–117.
8. Iglehart JK. Health insurers and medical-imaging policy–a work in progress. N Engl J Med 2009; 360:1030–1037.
9. Avorn J. Debate about funding comparative-effectiveness research. N Engl J Med 2009; 360:1927–1929.
10. Stern RG. Diagnostic imaging: powerful, indispensable, and out of control. Am J Med 2012; 125:113–114.
11. Donnelly LF. Reducing Radiation Dose Associated with Pediatric CT by Decreasing Unnecessary Examinations. Am. J. Roentgenol. 2005; 184:655–657.
12. Brenner DJ, Hall EJ. Computed tomography–an increasing source of radiation exposure. N Engl J Med 2007; 357:2277–2284.
13. Finkelstein EA, Trogdon JG, Cohen JW, Dietz W. Annual Medical Spending Attributable To Obesity: Payer- And Service-Specific Estimates. Health Aff (Millwood) 2009.
14. Kuppermann N, Holmes JF, Dayan PS, et al. Identification of children at very low risk of clinically-important brain injuries after head trauma: a prospective cohort study. Lancet 2009; 374:1160–1170.
15. Holmes JF, Wisner DH, McGahan JP, Mower WR, Kuppermann N. Clinical prediction rules for identifying adults at very low risk for intra-abdominal injuries after blunt trauma. Ann Emerg Med 2009; 54:575–584.
16. Slovis TL, Berdon WE. Panel discussion. Pediatric Radiology 2002; 32:242–244.
17. Brenner DJ, Hricak H. Radiation exposure from medical imaging: time to regulate? Jama 2010; 304:208–209.
18. Hendee WR, Becker GJ, Borgstede JP, et al. Addressing overutilization in medical imaging. Radiology 2010; 257:240–245.
19. Baicker K, Fisher ES, Chandra A. Malpractice liability costs and the practice of medicine in the Medicare program. Health Aff (Millwood) 2007; 26:841–852.
20. Dunnick NR, Applegate KE, Arenson RL. The inappropriate use of imaging studies: a report of the 2004 Intersociety Conference. J Am Coll Radiol 2005; 2:401–406.

21. Lehnert BE, Bree RL. Analysis of appropriateness of outpatient CT and MRI referred from primary care clinics at an academic medical center: how critical is the need for improved decision support? J Am Coll Radiol 2010; 7:192–197.

22. Miller RA, Sampson NR, Flynn JM. The prevalence of defensive orthopaedic imaging: a prospective practice audit in Pennsylvania. J Bone Joint Surg Am 2012; 94:e18.

23. Blachar A, Tal S, Mandel A, et al. Preauthorization of CT and MRI examinations: assessment of a managed care preauthorization program based on the ACR Appropriateness Criteria and the Royal College of Radiology guidelines. J Am Coll Radiol 2006; 3:851–859.

24. Sistrom CL, Dang PA, Weilburg JB, Dreyer KJ, Rosenthal DI, Thrall JH. Effect of computerized order entry with integrated decision support on the growth of outpatient procedure volumes: seven-year time series analysis. Radiology 2009; 251: 147–155.

25. X PRIZE Foundation and Qualcomm Foundation Set to Revolutionize Healthcare with Launch of $10 Million Qualcomm Tricorder X PRIZE. In:Medical Eletronic Device Solutions, 2012. Available online at: http://www.qualcommtricorderxprize.org/media/news-release/announcing-qualcomm-tricorder-x-prize [accessed February 20, 2013].

26. Institute of Medicine (U.S.). Committee on Breast Cancer and the Environment: The Scientific Evidence, Research Methodology, and Future Directions. Breast Cancer and the Environment: A Life Course Approach. In. Washington, DC: National Academy of Sciences, 2012; 469.

27. Elshaug AG, Bessen T, Moss JR, Hiller JE. Addressing "waste" in diagnostic imaging: some implications of comparative effectiveness research. J Am Coll Radiol 2010; 7:603–613.

28. Teasdale G, Jennett B. Assessment of coma and impaired consciousness. A practical scale. Lancet 1974; 2:81–84.

29. Centers for Disease Control and Prevention. Data collection of primary central nervous system tumors. National Program of Cancer Registries Training Materials. Atlanta, Georgia: Department of Health and Human Services, Centers for Disease Control and Prevention. 2004.

30. Heredia V, Ramalho M, Zapparoli M, Semelka RC. Incidence of pulmonary embolism and other chest findings in younger patients using multidetector computed tomography. Acta Radiol 2010; 51:402–406.

31. Venkatesh AK, Kline JA, Courtney DM, et al. Evaluation of Pulmonary Embolism in the Emergency Department and Consistency With a National Quality Measure: Quantifying the Opportunity for ImprovementEvaluation of Pulmonary Embolism in ER. Arch Intern Med 2012:1–5.

32. Srinivas SV, Deyo RA, Berger ZD. Application of "less is more" to low back pain. Arch Intern Med 2012; 172:1016–1020.

33. Deyo RA, Mirza SK, Martin BI. Back pain prevalence and visit rates: estimates from U.S. national surveys, 2002. Spine (Phila Pa 1976) 2006; 31:2724–2727.

34. Ivanova JI, Birnbaum HG, Schiller M, Kantor E, Johnstone BM, Swindle RW. Real-world practice patterns, health-care utilization, and costs in patients with low back pain: the long road to guideline-concordant care. Spine J 2011; 11:622–632.

35. Chou R, Fu R, Carrino JA, Deyo RA. Imaging strategies for low-back pain: systematic review and meta-analysis. Lancet 2009; 373:463–472.

36. Kendrick D, Fielding K, Bentley E, Kerslake R, Miller P, Pringle M. Radiography of the lumbar spine in primary care patients with low back pain: randomised controlled trial. Bmj 2001; 322:400–405.
37. The "top 5" lists in primary care: meeting the responsibility of professionalism. Arch Intern Med 2011; 171:1385–1390.
38. Webster BS, Cifuentes M. Relationship of early magnetic resonance imaging for work-related acute low back pain with disability and medical utilization outcomes. J Occup Environ Med 2010; 52:900–907.
39. Kanematsu M, Semelka RC, Leonardou P, et al. Angiogenesis in hepatocellular nodules: correlation of MR imaging and vascular endothelial growth factor. J Magn Reson Imaging 2004; 20:426–434.
40. Kanematsu M, Semelka RC, Leonardou P, Mastropasqua M, Lee JK. Hepatocellular carcinoma of diffuse type: MR imaging findings and clinical manifestations. J Magn Reson Imaging 2003; 18:189–195.
41. Karadeniz-Bilgili MY, Braga L, Birchard KR, et al. Hepatocellular carcinoma missed on gadolinium enhanced MR imaging, discovered in liver explants: retrospective evaluation. J Magn Reson Imaging 2006; 23:210–215.
42. Kelekis NL, Semelka RC, Worawattanakul S, et al. Hepatocellular carcinoma in North America: a multiinstitutional study of appearance on T1-weighted, T2-weighted, and serial gadolinium-enhanced gradient-echo images. AJR Am J Roentgenol 1998; 170:1005–1013.
43. Kierans AS, Leonardou P, Hayashi P, et al. MRI findings of rapidly progressive hepatocellular carcinoma. Magn Reson Imaging 2010; 28:790–796.
44. Mastropasqua M, Braga L, Kanematsu M, et al. Hepatic nodules in liver transplantation candidates: MR imaging and underlying hepatic disease. Magn Reson Imaging 2005; 23:557–562.
45. Shah TU, Semelka RC, Pamuklar E, et al. The risk of hepatocellular carcinoma in cirrhotic patients with small liver nodules on MRI. Am J Gastroenterol 2006; 101:533–540.
46. Tsurusaki M, Semelka RC, Uotani K, Sugimoto K, Fujii M, Sugimura K. Prospective comparison of high- and low-spatial-resolution dynamic MR imaging with sensitivity encoding (SENSE) for hypervascular hepatocellular carcinoma. Eur Radiol 2008; 18:2206–2212.
47. Patel MR, Peterson ED, Dai D, et al. Low diagnostic yield of elective coronary angiography. N Engl J Med 2010; 362:886–895.
48. Einstein AJ, Weiner SD, Bernheim A, et al. Multiple testing, cumulative radiation dose, and clinical indications in patients undergoing myocardial perfusion imaging. Jama 2010; 304:2137–2144.
49. Emanuel EJ. Cost savings at the end of life. What do the data show? Jama 1996; 275:1907–1914.
50. Jacobs P, Noseworthy TW. National estimates of intensive care utilization and costs: Canada and the United States. Crit Care Med 1990; 18:1282–1286.
51. Gilmer T, Schneiderman LJ, Teetzel H, et al. The costs of nonbeneficial treatment in the intensive care setting. Health Aff (Millwood) 2005; 24:961–971.

CHAPTER 3

Radiation dose reduction

Jorge Elias Jr[1] and Richard C. Semelka[2]
[1] The School of Medicine of Ribeirao Preto, University of Sao Paulo, Brazil
[2] University of North Carolina at Chapel Hill, School of Medicine, Department of Radiology, Chapel Hill, NC, USA

There is no doubt that we should be judicious in our use of radiation, ensuring that there is sufficient clinical benefit to radiation exposure. Deleterious side effects from radiation overexposure have been described in multiple reported series, with some of the most important reports in 2011 and 2012. Computed tomography (CT) applications using higher dose radiation, including positron emission tomography–CT (PET–CT), are increasing dramatically. Elimination of avoidable exposure to medical radiation is mandatory, independent of risks. Although disagreement exists regarding the extent of the risks of cancer from diagnostic X-ray methods, it is prudent to keep medical radiation exposure to "as low as reasonably achievable" (ALARA). In keeping with this imperative, CT manufacturers have made great strides in radiation-dose-controlling techniques over recent years.

Scope of the issue

X-rays: What are they?

X-rays are part of electromagnetic spectrum, with a wavelength situated between gamma rays and ultraviolet rays. Related to safety, in general terms the shorter the wavelength, the higher the energy deposition. X-rays are usually described in terms of their energy rather than wavelength, partly because of the very short wavelengths, and partly because energy deposition is the most critical factor in biological systems. It is also because X-rays tend to act more like particles than waveforms, for the purposes of

Health Care Reform in Radiology, First Edition. Richard C. Semelka and Jorge Elias Jr.
© 2013 John Wiley & Sons, Inc. Published 2013 by John Wiley & Sons, Inc.

imaging. X-rays can penetrate some solids, liquids, and all uncompressed gases. Gamma rays act in a similar way to X-rays, but they differ in their origin; X-rays are emitted by electrons outside the nucleus, whereas gamma rays are emitted by the nucleus.

All forms of ionization radiation are potentially hazardous. The biological effects of X-rays are categorized as stochastic and tissue reactive (previously termed deterministic). Tissue reactions happen when the dose exceeds a specific threshold and causes an immediate and predictable change to the tissue, classically observed as development of alopecia and a burning sensation, which increases over days and weeks and may culminate in ulcerative lesions. Cataract formation is another well-recognized tissue reaction effect. Stochastic effects include carcinogenic and genetic damage, considered to result from X-ray collisions with DNA, with resultant changes in DNA structure. Stochastic effects are considered to dominate in low exposure dose X-ray settings, with the net effects of damage not apparent until at least 2 years (sometimes 20 years or more) after the event.

German physicist Wilhelm Roentgen won the 1901 Nobel Prize in Physics for discovering X-rays in 1895, which gave birth over the ensuing decades to the profession of diagnostic radiology. X-rays, also known as roentgen rays, became a popular novelty in the early 1900s, bringing attention to many renowned scientists at that time, including Thomas Edison, who helped disseminate the technique. In the early days, injuries and casualties related to X-rays were largely ignored, although Roentgen's wife and Edison's assistant were two of the noteworthy early fatalities. Following the first 40–50 years after the discovery of X-rays, much would change regarding our knowledge of the effects and safety of these rays.

Lessons learned from the past

In August 1896, less than a year after Roentgen's discovery, the first account of skin damage was publicized. Since then, reports of injuries related to X-rays escalated. In those very early days, the administrators of X-rays had no instruments to measure the strength of the radiation and were unaware that large radiation doses could cause serious biological effects.

As a major sign of this era, a monument to the "radiation martyrs" was erected at St. George's Hospital in Hamburg in 1936 and had 159 names of X-ray victims engraved on it. Hundreds more have been added since. These X-ray martyrs were dedicated scientists, nurses, physicians, and technicians whose deaths in some ways have contributed to the knowledge of the field of Radiology. As brightly as the triumphs of science may shine, just as brightly burn the devastation of its mistakes [1].

Until the mid-1930s, approximately 200 radiologists had died as a result of radiation-induced malignant diseases (mainly leukemia). One of the earliest publications on the increased mortality from leukemia was reported in the *New England Journal of Medicine* (NEJM) [2]. Radiologists' shortened life-spans and causes of death took 50 years to come into alignment with those of other medical specialists. An essential change in radiation protection philosophy was developed at the first of The Tripartite Conferences on Radiation Protection, held in Ontario, Canada in 1949, with scientific and medical participants from the USA, Canada, and Great Britain. Contributions from that meeting included the assertions that "there may be some degree of risk at any level of exposure" and "the risk to the individual is not precisely determinable but however small is believed not to be zero."

On September 1, 1956 a landmark study by Giles et al. was the first to show that X-rays caused cancer in children of mothers who underwent medical X-rays during pregnancy [3]. This was a nationwide survey conducted by physicians throughout England, which demonstrated that pregnant women who received X-rays had a much greater likelihood that their children would develop leukemia than mothers who did not. Specifically, the study documented that 85 patients with leukemia had been exposed to radiation from maternal abdominal X-rays, while 45 patients did not have this prenatal exposure [3]. The authors concluded that "so large a total difference between the cases and controls can hardly be fortuitous" and that "the possibility that the peak of leukemia mortality noted by Hewitt [4] might be explained if weak irradiation could initiate changes in a fetus or very young child." They concluded that "this apparently harmless examination may occasionally cause leukemia or cancer in the unborn child."

This study created uproar at the time, but the findings were subsequently borne out in other surveys, including another large study that was conducted in the northeast USA. Yet these studies have been largely forgotten. Explanations for forgetting this lesson are manifold, including monetary reasons and lack of a distinctive group to keep this memory alive. Knowledge fades within 50 years, particularly if there is no perception that this knowledge has been deliberately or maliciously inflicted by another group. So with the passage of time and introduction of new exciting technology, it has been dropped from our conscious memory.

A follow-up review published in 1997 [5] considered that a causal explanation is supported by evidence indicating an appropriate dose–response relationship, in addition to findings established by animal experiments, and concluded that radiation doses on the order of 10 mGy (10 mSv) received by the fetus in utero produce a consequent increase in the risk of childhood cancer [5]. They reported that the excess absolute risk coefficient is approximately 6% per Gy of radiation exposure [5].

Radiation: Understanding what we are measuring and the risk controversies

The amount of energy deposited per unit of weight of human tissue is called the absorbed dose, which is measured using the System Internationale (SI) unit gray (Gy). The biological risk of the radiation exposure is measured using the SI unit sievert (Sv), which is the equivalent dose. Equal doses of all types of ionizing radiation are not equally harmful. Alpha particles produce greater harm than do beta particles, gamma rays and X-rays for a given absorbed dose. To account for this difference, radiation dose is expressed as equivalent dose in Sv. The dose in Sv is equal to "absorbed dose" multiplied by a "radiation weighting factor." The term "dose" or "radiation dose" generally refers to the equivalent dose.

Much that we have learned about the effects of radiation has come from the Hiroshima and Nagasaki bombings during World War II. There are many institutions that carry out ongoing investigations on this issue, including the Radiation Effects Research Foundation (RERF), a binational organization established in 1975, which was created and run by both the USA and Japan (formerly called the Atomic Bomb Casualty Commission).

No major scientific body that investigates radiation risks, including the International Commission on Radiological Protection (ICRP) [6], the National Academy of Sciences Committee on the Biological Effects of Ionizing Radiation (BEIR) [7], and the United Nations Scientific Committee on the Effects of Atomic Radiation (UNSCEAR) [8], recommends the use of a threshold dose for the induction of cancer. On January 31, 2005 the Department of Health and Human Services listed, for the first time, ionizing radiation as a known human carcinogen in the Eleventh Report on Carcinogens [9]. The most recent report on mortality from the Life Span Study (LSS) cohort of atom bomb survivors followed by the RERF shows that excess solid cancer risks appear to be linear in dose even for equivalent doses in the 0 to 150 mSv range, with no evidence for a threshold

[10]. In the USA, the National Council on Radiation Protection and Measurements recently concluded "that there is no conclusive evidence on which to reject the assumption of a linear-nonthreshold dose-response relationship for many of the risks attributable to low-level ionizing radiation" [11]. The results from the largest study of nuclear workers ever conducted showed radiation risks estimates that are "higher, but statistically compatible with, the risk estimates used for current radiation protection standards" [12].

The BEIR VII report, released in 2005 by the National Academy of Sciences, provides the most up-to-date and comprehensive risk estimates for cancer from exposure to low-level ionizing radiation. The BEIR VII executive summary states that "a comprehensive review of available biological and biophysical data supports a linear-no-threshold (LNT) risk model— that the risk of cancer proceeds in a linear fashion at lower doses without a threshold and that the smallest dose has the potential to cause a small increase in risk to humans" [13]. Low dose is defined by the BEIR VII committee as a dose in the range of near zero up to about 100 mSv (0.1 Sv). On average, assuming an age and sex distribution similar to that of the entire US population, the BEIR VII lifetime risk model predicts that approximately 1 individual in 1000 would develop cancer from an exposure to 10 mSv (0.01 Sv) of low dose radiation [13]. The BEIR VII report concludes by stating that future medical radiation studies are warranted and emphasizes that "of concern for radiological protection is the increasing use of computed tomography (CT) scans and diagnostic X rays" (www.nap.edu). It is therefore clear that the carcinogenic potential of radiation at doses encountered in CT needs to be taken seriously by the medical imaging community.

Nonetheless, it is important to recognize that there are considerable uncertainties in the current radiation risk estimates as provided by organizations such as the ICRP, UNSCEAR, and BEIR, especially at the lower dose levels encountered in CT [14]. The available evidence is not conclusive, primarily as a result of the absence of definitive epidemiological data at low dose levels. There are those who review the available epidemiological and radiobiological evidence, and conclude that the current ICRP risk estimates are too high [15–17]. It has also been suggested by the hormesis model that low dose radiation may be beneficial, and that our concerns with radiation risks at CT doses is unwarranted [18, 19]. Of note, the model of hormesis has been recently abandoned as unsubstantiated [20]. At the same time, it is also necessary to acknowledge that some have suggested that radiation risks may be even higher than those currently adopted for practical use by radiation protection bodies [21–23]. Organizations such as the Health Physics Society (2004) believe that the LNT is an oversimplification, and risk estimates should not be used at <50 mSv [24]. The French Academy of Sciences (2004) and American Nuclear Society (2001) hold that LNT overestimates risk [25, 26]. Radiation risk estimates at low radiation doses remains a controversial topic, and there is currently no scientific consensus regarding the existence of any threshold dose below which the risk of cancer induction would be zero.

Given the uncertainty as to whether there is, or is not, a threshold dose for radiation-induced cancer, any decision made may eventually turn out to be erroneous. If we assume there are radiation risks when there are none, we will be expending effort and resources to minimize nonexistent risks; however, if there truly are radiation risks that we choose to ignore, we will have subjected our patients to long-term detrimental consequences. Making decisions as to how to act in the presence of scientific uncertainty is essentially a political process, and therefore will require the use of value judgments [27].

Natural and artificial radiation exposure: A comparison

Naturally occurring "background" radiation exposure is omnipresent for every living being, as exposure to cosmic rays, inhalation of natural gas (radon), and intake of radioactive food and liquid occurs ubiquitously. We are exposed to radiation from natural sources all the time. According to recent estimates, the average person in the USA receives an effective dose of about 2.4 to 3 mSv per year from naturally occurring radioactive materials and cosmic radiation from outer space. These natural "background" doses vary between countries and within each country.

The added dose from cosmic rays during a coast-to-coast round-trip flight in a commercial airplane is about 0.03 mSv. Altitude plays an important role: with higher altitude there is greater exposure to cosmic rays. The largest source of background radiation (about 2 mSv per year) is radon gas, which is present in housing. Like other sources of background radiation, exposure to radon varies widely from one part of the country to another.

Medical radiation from X-rays and nuclear medicine is currently the largest artificial source of radiation exposure. The medical sources of radiation were about one-fifth of the natural radiation in 1987, close to half in 1993, and almost equivalent to natural radiation in 1997 in most affluent countries [28]. In 1997, the German Federal Office for Radiation Protection reported 136 million X-ray examinations and 4 million nuclear

Table 3.1 Natural and medical radiation doses (modified from [28, 29])

Source of exposure	Effective dose (mSv)
Natural radiation	**Per year**
Cosmic radiation	0.03
Rocks and soil	0.03
Naturally occurring radioactive material in the human body	0.04
Radon	2.00
Exposure to cosmic rays during a round-trip airplane flight from New York to Los Angeles	0.03
Diagnostic X-rays	**Per test**
Chest (PA film)	0.02
Limbs/joints	0.06
Head	0.07
Screening mammogram	0.13
Cervical spine	0.30
Abdomen	0.53
Pelvis/hip	0.83
Thoracic spine	1.40
Lumbar spine	1.80
Upper GI	3.60
Lower GI	6.40
CT	
Head	2.0
Abdomen*	10.0*
Chest*	20–40*
Pulmonary angiography*	20–40*
PET–CT	25
Interventional fluoroscopic procedures	25
Nuclear medicine	
Lung, renal, or thyroid scintigraphy	1
Bone scintigraphy	4
Thallium scan	23
Gallium scan	40

*CT protocols that overlap scanned regions or rescan the same anatomic region of interest, (e.g., noncontrasted and contrast-enhanced scans), impart two to three times the radiation dose.

medicine diagnostic tests, resulting in a mean effective dose of 2.15 mSv per person per year [28]. Some examples of natural and medical radiation doses are presented in Table 3.1.

As shown in Table 3.1, the effective dose of most diagnostic X-ray examinations is low. Nonetheless, virtually all scientific studies published on this subject have shown an elevated risk for the development of cancer in patients exposed to diagnostic X-rays. In a retrospective cohort study by Morin Doody et al. reviewing 5573 female patients with scoliosis, the authors concluded that these young patients exposed to serial radiographic examinations showed a relative risk of 1.6 for breast cancer for an average dose of 108 mSv [30]. Two interesting aspects of this study are that it described the cumulative risk factor of multiple repeat radiation exposures, and that young female patients are a particularly high radiation-sensitive risk group.

The greatest contributor to this dramatic increase in population medical radiation exposure is CT scans [31]. In the USA, annual CT examinations are now approaching 80 million and increasing by approximately 10% per year [32]. The Food and Drug Administration (FDA) estimates that a CT examination with an effective dose of 10 mSv, or one CT of the abdomen, may be associated with an increased chance of developing fatal cancer for approximately one individual in 2000, whereas the BEIR VII lifetime risk model predicts that with the same low dose radiation, approximately 1 individual in 1000 will develop cancer [13, 33]. The difference appears to be the use of the term 'fatal' in the FDA estimate. Compared with the overall risk to the individual for developing cancer—approximately 42 per 100 individuals—imaging-based radiation risk may appear small. However, from a public health risk perspective, this small individual cancer risk must be multiplied by a large and ever-increasing population of individuals undergoing CT examinations [13, 29]. Estimates suggest that approximately 29,000 future cancers could be related to CT scan use in the USA in 2007 alone [34].

CT radiation doses are much higher than conventional radiography doses. For instance, one chest CT scan involves an effective dose anywhere from 100 to 1000 times greater than that from a corresponding chest radiograph [35]. The relatively high radiation dose of CT examinations when compared with other medical imaging studies is further compounded by the common ordering practice of multiple CT examinations on the same patient. In a large cohort, retrospective analysis spanning two decades, 33% of patients underwent five or more CT studies [36]. Such practice results in cumulative CT radiation exposure, and adds incrementally to baseline cancer risk [36]. Additionally, in a recent multi-institutional analysis of radiation dose associated with common CT examinations in the San Francisco Bay Area, California, there was substantial variation in doses within and between institutions with a 13-fold variation between the highest and lowest dose for identical CT procedures [37]. Hence, depending on where and when an individual receives a CT study, the effective dose received could substantially exceed the median.

The pediatric population represents a particularly vulnerable group of individuals at increased risk for cancer [38]. A 1-year-old infant is 10–15 times more likely than a 50-year-old adult to develop a malignancy for the same dose of radiation [39]. Children are at greater risk than adults from a given dose of radiation because of enhanced radiosensitivity of developing tissues and more remaining years of life during which a radiation-induced cancer could develop [40]. Despite the evidence of known cancer risks for CT-related radiation, the number of pediatric CT studies performed annually in the USA is 7 million [41].

Some of the most compelling data on the deleterious effect of radiation from current medical imaging (CT and advanced angiography) have been published in the last couple of years. Eisenberg et al. reported from a large population study in Quebec, Canada that for every 10 mSv of low dose ionizing radiation, there was a 3% increase in the risk of age- and sex-adjusted cancer over a mean follow-up period of 5 years, in a population of 82,861 patients [42]. In the 10-year follow-up period in total 12,020 incident cancers were diagnosed, confirming a dose-dependent relationship between exposure to radiation from cardiac procedures and subsequent risk of cancer [42]. Moreover, Eisenberg et al. showed that cumulative exposure from cardiac procedures is an independent predictor of incident cancer (hazard ratio [HR] 1.003 per mSv, 95% confidence interval [CI] 1.002–1.004) [42]. This study represented the first large-scale study to directly show that CT resulted in cancer. In an even more current study, Pearce et al. observed that CT scans in children that deliver a cumulative dose of about 50 mGy may triple the risk of leukemia and doses of about 60 mGy may triple the risk of brain cancer [43]. However, because these cancers are relatively rare, the cumulative absolute risks are small; in the 10 years after the first scan for patients younger than 10 years, one excess case of leukemia and one excess case of brain tumor per 10,000 head CT scans is estimated to occur [43]. The comparison with the LSS of Japanese atom bomb survivors [44] presented by the authors is striking. The dose–response for leukemia following childhood exposure and similar follow-up time (<15 years after exposure) in the LSS was 0.045 per mSv, which was comparable to the estimate they derived [43]. For brain tumors, their result was about four times higher than the LSS estimate (0.0061 per mSv [0.0001–0.0639] <20 years after exposure) [43].

Although financial incentive by fee-for-service environments is a major driver for overuse of CT scanning, a comparable explosive growth has also been observed in large integrated health care systems [45]. A recent published retrospective analysis of electronic records of members of six large integrated systems from different regions of the USA has shown a substantial increase in the rate of advanced diagnostic imaging and associated radiation exposure between 1996 and 2010 [45]. In particular, the increased use of CT between 1996 and 2010 resulted in a doubled mean per capita effective dose (1.2 mSv versus 2.3 mSv), and the proportion of patients who received high (>20–50 mSv) exposure (1.2 versus 2.5%) and very high (>50 mSv) annual radiation exposure (0.6 versus 1.4%) also increased greatly [45]. Presumably this reflects the perception of the importance of keeping up with the general practice of medicine in academic and private practice situations—the medical equivalent of "keeping up with the Joneses."

Ideal solution

The ideal solution would be to replace all ionizing radiation-based imaging methods, namely X-rays, CTs, and nuclear medicine studies, with those that do not utilize ionizing radiation—ultrasound and magnetic resonance imaging (MRI) primarily—and to return to the approach in former years of relying on good clinical acumen to make therapeutic decisions for patients. Unfortunately, regarding clinical acumen, retracing the steps of the past are difficult, as expectations by physicians and patients are somewhat entrenched, compounded by the concerns of medical litigation. General replacement of ionizing radiation-based studies by ultrasound, MRI, and future imaging methods is feasible but probably a very slow process. Furthermore, these ionizing and non-ionizing imaging methods are complementary with each other in some clinical settings, and in a number of medical scenarios (notably chest disease and major trauma) the strengths of CT imaging are unmatched. Moreover, far from being replaced, these X-ray based methods have increasing clinical applications, as now is occurring with PET–CT.

Workable solution

In the absence of definitive evidence on the effects of low dose radiation, and a corresponding consensus in the scientific community, the prudent course of action is to act on the assumption that low dose radiation may well cause cancer. If we assume that X-ray imaging radiation doses may cause cancer, it would be reasonable for the radiology community to seek ways to eliminate unnecessary radiation exposure while ensuring appropriate utilization of these methods. An X-ray based method, including CT examination, may be considered indicated when the benefits of the study would outweigh any assumed radiation risks. Adoption of this course of action would not be expected to impede the undoubted benefits of technology for all indicated examinations.

Current investigation is now ongoing to investigate various strategies that result in reductions, at times dramatic, in the dose of radiation delivered by CT, resulting in decreases of radiation from 10 mSv or greater, to potentially substantially less than 1 mSv. Techniques such as modulation of the delivery of X-rays based on tissue thickness, post-processing modeling methodologies, and tailored kVp applications are either established or en route to being practical for clinical use—this may result in many CT scans delivering <1 mSv of radiation per study, which will be less than we propose as the cut-off value for when informed consent should be employed when recommending an imaging study to a subject (see Chapter 5).

Conclusions

In summary, regardless of what the exciting future may hold, essential components of an effective strategy to promote patient safety and minimize any detrimental effects of radiation exposures would encompass the following:
- perform only X-rays studies that are needed (Chapter 1);
- consider alternatives to X-ray based methods, mainly to CT (Chapter 4);
- keep patient doses ALARA;
- improve education and communication to the medical staff and patients (Chapter 5).

References

1. Evans J. The Clarity of Night. The Martyrs, Part 3. Available online at: http://clarityofnight.blogspot.com.br/2006/03/martyrs-part-3.html [accessed February 25, 2013].
2. Ulrich H. Incidence of leukemia in radiologists. New Engl J Med 1946; 234: 742–743.

3. Giles D, Hewitt D, Stewart A, Webb J. Malignant disease in childhood and diagnostic irradiation in utero. Lancet 1956; 271:447.

4. Hewitt D. Some features of leukaemia mortality. Br J Prev Soc Med 1955; 9:81–88.

5. Doll R, Wakeford R. Risk of childhood cancer from fetal irradiation. Br J Radiol 1997; 70:130–139.

6. 1990 Recommendations of the International Commission on Radiological Protection. Ann ICRP 1991; 21:1–201.

7. Committee on the Biological Effects of Ionizing Radiation (BEIR V) NRC. Health Effects of Exposure to Low Levels of Ionizing Radiation: BEIR V. Washington, DC: National Academy Press, 1990.

8. United Nations Scientific Committee on the Effects of Atomic Radiation, 2000. UNSCEAR 2000 Report to the General Assembly.

9. National Toxicology Program NTP. 11th Report on Carcinogens. Research Triangle Park, NC: The Department of Health and Human Services, 2005.

10. Preston DL, Shimizu Y, Pierce DA, Suyama A, Mabuchi K. Studies of mortality of atomic bomb survivors. Report 13: Solid cancer and noncancer disease mortality: 1950–1997. Radiat Res 2003; 160:381–407.

11. Evaluation of the Linear-Nonthreshold Dose-Response Model for Ionizing Radiation (2001). Report no. 136. Bethesda, MD: The National Council on Radiation Protection and Measurements (NCRP), 2001.

12. Cardis E, Vrijheid M, Blettner M, et al. Risk of cancer after low doses of ionising radiation: retrospective cohort study in 15 countries. BMJ 2005; 331:77.

13. Committee on the Biological Effects of Ionizing Radiation (BEIR V) NRC. Executive Summary. Health Risks from Exposure to Low Levels of Ionizing Radiation: BEIR VII Phase 2. Washington, D.C.: National Academy Press, 2005.

14. Uncertainties in Fatal Cancer Risk Estimates Used in Radiation Protection (1997). Report no. 126. Bethesda, MD: The National Council on Radiation Protection and Measurements (NCRP), 1997.

15. Cohen BL. Cancer risk from low-level radiation. AJR Am J Roentgenol 2002; 179:1137–1143.

16. Romerio F. Which paradigm for managing the risk of ionizing radiation? Risk Anal 2002; 22:59–66.

17. Rossi HH, Zaider M. Radiogenic lung cancer: The effects of low doses of low linear energy transfer (LET) radiation. Radiat Environ Biophys 1997; 36:85–88.

18. Sagan LA. What is hormesis and why haven't we heard about it before? Special Issue on Radiation Hormesis. Health Phys 1987; 52:517–680.

19. Cameron JR, Moulder JE. Proposition: Radiation hormesis should be elevated to a position of scientific respectability. Med Phys 1998; 25:1407–1410.

20. The 2007 Recommendations of the International Commission on Radiological Protection. Publication 103. Ann ICRP 2007; 37:1–332.

21. Gofman JW. Radiation and Human Health. San Francisco, CA: Sierra Club Books, 1981.

22. Kneale GW, Stewart AM. Reanalysis of Hanford data: 1944–1986 deaths. Am J Ind Med 1993; 23:371–389.

23. Ehrle LH. Ionising radiation in infancy and adult cognitive function: Much research on low dose radiation remains hidden. BMJ 2004; 328:582; author reply 582.

24. Radiation risk in perspective: Position statement of the Health Physics Society. McLean, VA: Health Physics Society, 2004.

25. Health effects of low-level radiation: Position statement. La Grange Park, IL: American Nuclear Society, 2001.

26. Thé G, Tubiana M. Irradiation médicale, déchets, désinformation: Un avis de l'Académie de médecine. Bull Acad Natle Méd 2001; 185:1671–1680.

27. Brunk CG, Haworth L, Lee B. Value assumptions in risk assessment. Waterloo, Ontario: Wilfrid Laurier University Press, 1991.

28. Picano E. Sustainability of medical imaging. BMJ 2004; 328:578–580.

29. Semelka RC, Armao DM, Elias J, Jr., Huda W. Imaging strategies to reduce the risk of radiation in CT studies, including selective substitution with MRI. J Magn Reson Imaging 2007; 25:900–909.

30. Morin Doody M, Lonstein JE, Stovall M, Hacker DG, Luckyanov N, Land CE. Breast cancer mortality after diagnostic radiography: Findings from the U.S. Scoliosis Cohort Study. Spine 2000; 25:2052–2063.

31. Mettler FA, Jr., Bhargavan M, Faulkner K, et al. Radiologic and nuclear medicine studies in the United States and worldwide: Frequency, radiation dose, and comparison with other radiation sources—1950–2007. Radiology 2009; 253:520–531.

32. Brenner DJ, Hricak H. Radiation exposure from medical imaging: Time to regulate? JAMA 2010; 304:208–209.

33. U.S. Food and Drug Administration. What are the Radiation Risks from CT? Available online at: http://www.fda.gov/ForConsumers/ConsumerUpdates/ucm115329.htm [accessed February 25, 2013].

34. Berrington de Gonzalez A, Mahesh M, Kim KP, et al. Projected cancer risks from computed tomographic scans performed in the United States in 2007. Arch Intern Med 2009; 169:2071–2077.

35. Picano E, Vano E. The radiation issue in cardiology: the time for action is now. Cardiovasc Ultrasound 2011; 9:35.

36. Sodickson A, Baeyens PF, Andriole KP, et al. Recurrent CT, cumulative radiation exposure, and associated radiation-induced cancer risks from CT of adults. Radiology 2009; 251:175–184.

37. Smith-Bindman R, Lipson J, Marcus R, et al. Radiation dose associated with common computed tomography examinations and the associated lifetime attributable risk of cancer. Arch Intern Med 2009; 169:2078–2086.

38. Dixon AK, Dendy P. Spiral CT: How much does radiation dose matter? Lancet 1998; 352:1082–1083.

39. Hall EJ. Lessons we have learned from our children: Cancer risks from diagnostic radiology. Pediatr Radiol 2002; 32:700–706.

40. Brenner DJ, Hall EJ. Computed tomography—an increasing source of radiation exposure. N Engl J Med 2007; 357:2277–2284.

41. Shah NB, Platt SL. ALARA: Is there a cause for alarm? Reducing radiation risks from computed tomography scanning in children. Curr Opin Pediatr 2008; 20:243–247.

42. Eisenberg MJ, Afilalo J, Lawler PR, Abrahamowicz M, Richard H, Pilote L. Cancer risk related to low-dose ionizing radiation from cardiac imaging in patients after acute myocardial infarction. CMAJ 2011; 183:430–436.

43. Pearce MS, Salotti JA, Little MP, et al. Radiation exposure from CT scans in childhood and subsequent risk of leukaemia and brain tumours: A retrospective cohort study. Lancet 2012; 380: 499–505.

44. Preston DL, Kusumi S, Tomonaga M, et al. Cancer incidence in atomic bomb survivors. Part III. Leukemia, lymphoma and multiple myeloma, 1950–1987. Radiat Res 1994; 137:S68–97.

45. Smith-Bindman R, Miglioretti DL, Johnson E, et al. Use of diagnostic imaging studies and associated radiation exposure for patients enrolled in large integrated health care systems, 1996-2010. JAMA 2012; 307:2400–2409.

CHAPTER 4

Alternate imaging studies to CT

Jorge Elias Jr,[1] Lauren M. B. Burke,[2] and Richard C. Semelka[2]

[1]The School of Medicine of Ribeirao Preto, University of Sao Paulo, Brazil
[2]University of North Carolina at Chapel Hill, School of Medicine, Department of Radiology, Chapel Hill, NC, USA

The use of magnetic resonance imaging (MRI) and ultrasound (US) avoids exposure to ionizing radiation encountered in computed tomography (CT), and may be appropriately substituted for a wide range of clinical indications. Yet, to the present time, because of the ease of performance, the speed, and the relative ease of interpretation of CT, there has been a continued expansion in its utilization. This is despite the well-vocalized concerns of excess use of medical ionizing radiation.

Scope of the issue

Medical imaging: The role in modern medicine through evidence-based research

Medical imaging has transformed health care delivery through its substantial impact on disease prevention, early detection, diagnosis, and treatment. Oftentimes modern medical imaging and CT are used interchangeably, which is a practice that we believe should be separated, and is part of the substance of this chapter. Many physicians advocate that with CT imaging patient outcomes are improved and costs are reduced. This is likely correct, although confirmatory studies are sparse and it is difficult to confirm validity of the endpoints of the data that have been published. Not surprisingly, this is not exclusive for CT imaging, as it has been clear that controversies exist about mammography screening for breast cancer. The mortality reduction due to mammography screening in eight randomized trials ranges from 0% to 32% [1]. In fact, recently Woloshin and Schwartz

Health Care Reform in Radiology, First Edition. Richard C. Semelka and Jorge Elias Jr.
© 2013 John Wiley & Sons, Inc. Published 2013 by John Wiley & Sons, Inc.

opined that the timing of breast cancer diagnosis has minimal impact on long-term survival, citing evidence that mammography reduces a 50-year-old woman's 10-year risk of dying of breast cancer from 0.53% to 0.46% [2]. Additionally, in mammography, as in CT, overdiagnosis should be a concern, as it can sometimes do more harm than good, but this often goes unmentioned in public messages about mammography [3–6]. Nonetheless, it does appear a rational assumption that if the patient receives the correct study for the clinical indication, and in a timely fashion, that patients benefit, and health care dollars are saved. It may also be a reasonable assertion by the *New England Journal of Medicine* that medical imaging is one of the top "developments that changed the face of clinical medicine" during the last millennium [7].

Although the accumulated literature regarding medical imaging through scientific and evidence-based research is extensive, though often with limitations, as we mention above, such as appropriate endpoints, the rapid development of new techniques and new applications pose yet another challenge to update and keep current evaluations of the roles of various imaging modalities and their comparative effectiveness. Clearly it is an important part of modern health care to continuously maintain current imaging strategies, to reevaluate standard approaches in light of new developments, and to replace older, perhaps less accurate and/or less safe, approaches with newer techniques that are more beneficial to patients and society. Each diagnostic test has a complement of characteristics that reflect the results expected to be accomplished in patients with and without disease [8]. No diagnostic test is perfect, and there are always flaws that must be acknowledged, understood, and managed. There is usually an overlap of test results among patients, with and without a specific disease, that result in healthy individuals occasionally being classified wrongly as diseased, and some diseased individuals failing to be detected. Study data documenting the extent to which a test result accurately reflects reality can be analyzed in several ways [8]. In order to improve the accuracy and completeness of reporting imaging studies, most experts recommend standardization strategies, such as the Standards for Reporting of Diagnostic Accuracy (STARD) [9, 10] and the Consolidated Standards of Reporting Trials (CONSORT) [11], as has been reported in randomized controlled trials studies.

The complexity inherent in the evaluation of efficacy of a diagnostic imaging test is staggering and was described in a publication by Fryback and Thornbury in 1991 [12], who proposed a six-level hierarchical model of efficacy comprising technical efficacy, diagnostic accuracy efficacy, diagnostic thinking efficacy, therapeutic efficacy, patient outcome efficacy, and societal efficacy. A perfect diagnostic test would be technically feasible, easy to obtain, have 100% accuracy, affect the clinician's diagnostic understanding of the patient's disease, determine therapy both by indicating certain or preventing other procedures and/or medical treatments, result in clinical improvement of patients while diminishing morbidity and mortality, and finally would meet criteria for analyses in cost–benefit, cost–effectiveness, and cost–utility. Research tools have been developed to achieve these types of analyses, and resource centers have been created to help in the search and organization of these; one noteworthy example is The Cochrane Library (www.thecochranelibrary.com).

The case of CT: More and faster translates into better health? Radiation dose aside, the need for more evidence-based research

There is no doubt that CT has resulted in a profound change in medicine, beginning in the last decades of the 20th century. It seems clear that CT's usefulness is well-established for some clinical indications; the evidence is more controversial for many others. A common refrain made in defense of CT, in the face of concerns of overutilization and radiation risks, is that CT has saved thousands of lives. But where is the evidence or the study to show this? This statement appears authoritative, but is not based on a real foundation. A more factually correct statement, although lacking in dramatic public appeal, is that in a number of clinical circumstances the information from CT has likely contributed substantially to the appropriate management of patients, which has most likely improved their outcomes and longevity. CT is the modality best able to evaluate major trauma, and is at present not substitutable by MRI or US, especially where the major trauma involves or includes the thorax. There is no substitute for CT in the evaluation of injuries or disease processes that involve air localization in abnormal spaces. Controversy enters this assessment when trauma is of variable severity; the more severe the trauma, the more CT is beneficial and likely imperative—the less severe the trauma, the less the importance of CT. Unfortunately it is difficult to tease out severity in most studies that have made these evaluations in trauma patients, which is why some studies show value to CT and others not so much [13–15]. In other clinical situations where CT is widely praised, such as the detection of major vascular crises, such as aortic type-A dissections, or major arterial thrombosis, where their detection may indeed be life-saving, studies or commentaries that have advocated the importance of CT in this setting have usually been performed in isolation, with no assessment of comparative effectiveness in relation to MRI [16–18]. Many of these determinations can be made with approximately the same accuracy with MRI, without the downsides of medical radiation and iodine-based contrast-induced nephropathy (CIN). In our clinical experience in patients who are stable and cooperative, MRI can perform as well as CT in large and medium-sized vessel disease.

One good example of the controversy of the use of CT in a clinical situation is CT use in acute appendicitis. As radiologists, we intrinsically believe that an important disease that can be life threatening and can be detected by imaging should be detected by imaging. Some studies have not shown that detection by CT imaging has resulted in benefit [19]. A further confounding aspect is that imaging in acute appendicitis is generally considered a CT domain; whereas it is clear that in pediatrics, US performs well in this setting, and in all patients, a well-performed and well-interpreted MRI is likely as good or perhaps better [20–22]. Some studies have reported that the increased use of preoperative imaging and laparoscopy has had no impact on clinical outcomes in patients undergoing appendectomy [23]. This particular study showed that the significant increase in the use of preoperative imaging and laparoscopy in the management of patients with acute appendicitis in more recent years, compared with earlier years, failed to reduce the negative appendectomy, perforation, and complication rates [23]. Another recent study showed that the increasing use of CT scanning in acute appendicitis has increased the cost of care, decreased the contribution to overall benefit, prolonged the patient's stay in the emergency department, and delayed the time to operation [24]. In contrast, a recently published meta-analysis supports the hypothesis that the use of preoperative abdominal CT is associated with lower negative appendectomy rates [25]. The position of these authors is that although the use of CT in the absence of an expedited imaging protocol may delay surgery, this delay is not associated with increased appendiceal perforation rates, and they conclude that routine CT in all patients presenting with suspected appendicitis could reduce the rate of unnecessary surgery without increasing morbidity [25]. The upshot of correlating these studies is that there is considerable controversy about the value of CT imaging for appendicitis, even ignoring radiation and CIN. Skeptically, one cannot ignore the observation that physicians who do not benefit financially from the use of CT are apt to come out against its use, whereas those who do benefit generally observe the opposite findings. We believe though, that taking a measured prudent look, in the setting where a physician has performed a physical examination and has a strong clinical suspicion for acute appendicitis, that imaging is beneficial. CT does work well and is fast, but it would be appropriate to use US in place of CT in children, if the appropriate experience by US-trained radiologists is present; and similarly MRI should be considered in many subjects, again if the expertise is present. If the expertise is not present, it should be developed. Many centers, including our own, have adopted the use of noncontrast MRI to evaluate for acute appendicitis in pregnant patients [20, 26, 27]. We believe this role for MRI should be considerably expanded into children and young adults as a whole.

On the other hand, there is no controversy about the accuracy of noncontrast helical CT for the diagnosis of urolithiasis [28–30]. Unfortunately, because of its undisputed ability to demonstrate renal stones, renal stone CT has become one of the most overused indications, and it is not uncommon that in many studies that evaluate overuse, noncontrast CT for renal stones is one of the greatest culprits, with CTs repeated in excess of five times per year consistently reported [31]. This overuse of CT in this setting unquestioningly has little to no patient benefit, with probably considerable likelihood of harm.

In a similar fashion, CT pulmonary angiography (CTPA) has been shown to be highly accurate for the diagnosis of pulmonary embolism (PE), and has become the first-line imaging modality for the assessment of this clinical indication, as it evaluates the pulmonary arterial vasculature well, including subsegmental branches [32, 33]. Unfortunately, because of its success, CT is vastly overused for this clinical indication. Heredia et al. reported that in young females only 5% of subjects examined with CT for PE actually had PE [34]. This overuse of CT in this setting has generated great concern, especially in younger adults, and particularly because of the risks for the development of breast cancer in young women, due to the high sensitivity to radiation damage of younger breast tissue [35]. In response to the concerns of radiation risk, gadolinium-enhanced 3D gradient-echo sequence has been developed and proposed as an alternative technique for the visualization of central, lobar, and segmental arteries, and may diagnose PE and other pathologies involving the chest in a variety of patient populations, as no radiation is involved with this approach [36]. It should be noted, that up to the present time MRI cannot adequately assess interstitial lung disease and related processes, and these remain the domain of CT [37, 38].

It has been reported that high-quality CT imaging results in shorter hospital stays and also faster onset of appropriate medical care and therapy

[39]. Although this is likely true, our opinion is that this relates to modern imaging in general, and not to CT specifically, and imaging trends should be toward MRI/US rather than CT [40]. We advocate that for abdominal and pelvic imaging, US and MRI are safer alternatives to CT in many cases. For most clinical problems in which CT is used, MRI would provide an acceptable or preferred alternative [41]. In many disease settings, MRI is underused, which in part reflects the antiquated knowledge and experience of older referring physicians and radiologists. Much of the perception of why MRI should not be used is based on outdated thinking of saving health care dollars, which is based on older literature, and suppositions, rather than current knowledge. Cost and speed of examination for MRI has been improving and continues to improve, although expertise has been lagging [40]; this too is continuing to improve, as more younger generation radiologists are trained to be proficient in MRI.

When and why to choose MRI?

MRI has become a well-established imaging method, reflecting the rapid pace of technological advances, and more widespread knowledge and education among physicians and radiologists. Advances over the last decade and longer include:

1. remote movement of the imaging table from the imaging console;
2. multiple input channels that allow simultaneous use of multiple localized, specialized surface coils that generate high-resolution (high image quality) images of multiple regions of the body, without the delay of coil exchange and setup;
3. specialized surface coils that are designed for independent operation of the individual coil elements;
4. concurrent development of sequence (data acquisition) technology that operates in conjunction with the new specialized coils, such as parallel imaging and radial acquisition;
5. development of high image quality 3D T1-weighted gradient echo and radial acquisition imaging, with short echo time (TE), that facilitates acceptable imaging quality of various organ systems in which motion is a problem—most notably the lungs.

The combined effect of all of these innovations has allowed, among other things, whole-body imaging to be performed more rapidly (because of remote table movement and new short data acquisitions), with maintenance of high image quality (simultaneous use of multiple specialized coils), and with the ability to image the lungs with adequate image quality (3D T1-weighted gradient echo imaging, radial acquisition imaging). The

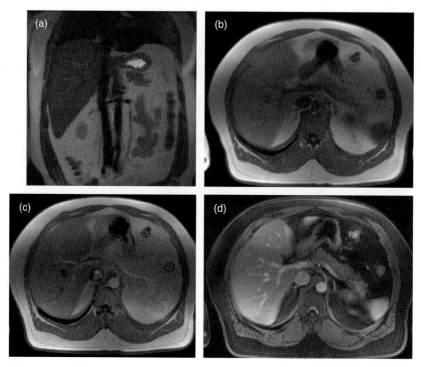

Figure 4.1 Whole-body MRI study of the abdominal region. (a) Coronal T2-weighted fat-suppressed, single-shot echo train spin echo; axial T1-weigthed 2D gradient-echo (b) unenhanced and (c) gadolinium-enhanced on hepatic arterial dominant phase; and (d) axial gadolinium-enhanced 3D fat-suppressed gradient echo.

net effect is that the entire body can be imaged in a matter of 10–15 minutes, with high image quality maintained (Figure 4.1 to 4.4).

MRI is an imaging modality that is considerably safer than CT on the basis of a number of factors, of which radiation exposure is perhaps the most serious and most discussed. In addition, MRI is much more accurate in detecting disease in many settings. Although MRI is recognized to be superior to CT in a number of organ systems, a pivotal article also has shown that screening MRI of the entire body may be as accurate or more accurate than individual "gold-standard" diagnostic investigations of individual organ systems [42]. The accuracy of modern MRI to evaluate the full range of organ systems should cause reevaluation of how different imaging investigations should be used to ensure the welfare of patients and optimize their care.

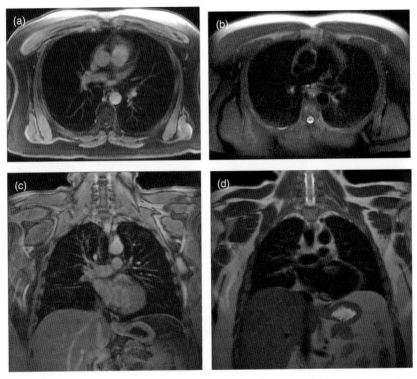

Figure 4.2 Whole-body MRI study of the thoracic region. Axial (a) and (b) coronal T1-weighted fat-suppressed 3D gradient echo; axial (c) and (d) coronal T2-weighted fat-suppressed, single-shot echo train spin echo.

Up to now, MRI has often been thought of as an alternative to CT investigation, either in patients who have contraindications to CT (allergy to contrast agents or poor renal function) or in whom CT findings are considered inconclusive. The prudent approach for the future may be a change in the paradigm of imaging investigation to less harmful techniques, with the preferential use of US or MRI when accuracy of these techniques is approximately equivalent to CT, and CT reserved as a problem-solving modality and for those indications in which CT is clearly superior.

Of particular importance is the pediatric patient, a population in which radiation exposure is directed at developing organs that are extremely radiosensitive, or breast tissue in female children and women. Examples of circumstances where imaging studies are often repeated, and hence

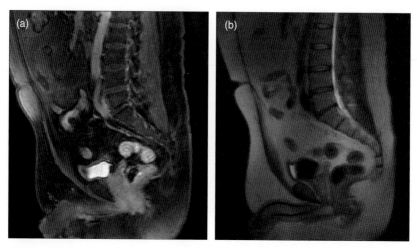

Figure 4.3 Whole-body MRI study of the pelvic region. (a) Sagittal T1-weighted fat-suppressed 3D gradient echo; and (b) T2-weighted echo-train spin echo.

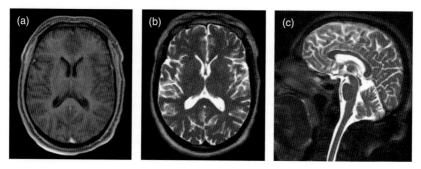

Figure 4.4 Whole-body MRI study of the head. (a) Axial T1-weighted fat-suppressed 3D gradient echo; and axial (b) and sagittal (c) T2-weighted fat-suppressed single-shot echo train spin echo.

preferential use of safer imaging strategies is prudent, include patients with Crohn's disease or of childhood abdominal malignancies, such as Wilms' tumor or neuroblastoma. The "image gently" physician and patient awareness campaign was specifically established by the combined efforts of radiologic and pediatric societies in order to develop safer approaches to image children [43–45].

For many neurologic and musculoskeletal applications, the evolution of MRI to replace CT has largely taken place. MRI is certainly the mainstay for diseases or injuries that involve soft tissues such as muscle and cartilage, and MRI is superior for the evaluation of medullary bone. By contrast, for anatomical delineation of cortical bone, in particular in the setting of major trauma and major fractures in complex joints, CT is the appropriate tool.

In the abdomen, the hallmark example of the superiority of MRI over CT is liver lesion and diffuse liver disease evaluation. Currently, a logical early step in transitioning imaging investigation to safer, more accurate approaches would be to perform MRI as the primary imaging tool to investigate diseases of the liver. The rationale for this is fourfold: 1) the intrinsic safety of the modality, the contrast agents, and the intravenous injection process (attention must be paid to nephrogenic systemic fibrosis); 2) the established greater accuracy of MRI over CT in liver investigation [46]; 3) the ease of performing these studies; and 4) the ease of interpreting these studies, even without extensive MRI training. A number of practices by various radiology agencies would need to be modified to aid in this conversion, including recommendations by the American College of Radiology and increasing the content of abdominal MRI examination material on the American Board of Radiology certification examinations.

The pancreas is another organ in which MRI is often superior to CT in detecting disease—in particular for the most important disease of the pancreas, the small pancreatic ductal carcinoma. In patients who can follow breath-holding instructions MRI is vastly superior [46–52]. This is of critical importance, as small pancreatic cancers are difficult to impossible to see on CT (but well shown on MRI), and pancreatic cancer grows quickly while being the most lethal of the 10 commonest cancers (pancreatic cancer at number 5). If detected when it is less than 1 cm in size and surgically excised, patients may experience normal longevity [53], rather than the 5%, 5-year survival traditionally reported for pancreatic cancer. Survival for pancreatic cancer has not changed substantially in decades, despite the development of modern therapies. Although MRI is able to visualize pancreatic cancers that are less than 1 cm in diameter, the current challenge is an inability to identify subjects who are at high risk of pancreatic cancer [53], as often when patients become symptomatic from the disease, the disease has already become incurable. Pancreatic islet cell tumors, the second most common malignancies of the pancreas, are also vastly better shown on MRI than CT [49, 54, 55].

Beyond the liver and pancreas, the majority of benign, malignant, and inflammatory diseases of the abdomen and pelvis are well shown on MRI, and in the hands of experienced practitioners, are better elucidated than on CT; these include diseases of the spleen, adrenals, kidneys, pancreas, and male and female pelvis. The kidneys, adrenal glands, and spleen show slight advantages in diagnostic accuracy for MRI in comparison with CT. Yet CT is often done instead, reflecting the perception that the differences are minimal, CT is slightly less expensive, CT studies can generally be acquired sooner, and physicians have more familiarity with CT images. In the proposed new imaging paradigm, many of these patients should undergo MRI. MRI is only marginally superior diagnostically to CT; however, it is safer and therefore should be used preferentially.

Imaging of bowel diseases poses challenges for both CT and MRI, and with some conditions CT is superior and with others MRI is superior, from a diagnostic accuracy point of view. Taking safety into consideration, MRI probably should be performed in patients who need to undergo multiple repeat studies (e.g. patients with Crohn's disease).

The evaluation of vessel disease with imaging studies requires comparison of the relative strengths of MR angiography (MRA) and CT angiography (CTA) to be weighed, with the additional consideration that both techniques continue to undergo rapid improvement, so continual reassessment is important. MRA is excellent for large and medium sized vessels, and because of safety considerations should be used to study diseases of these vessels (e.g. the abdominal aorta or carotid arteries). Because of the higher spatial resolution of CT (i.e. it can acquire thinner sections), small vessels are currently better studied by CT; an excellent example of this is coronary CTA (imaging the arteries in the heart). Over the last decade, the greater speed of data acquisition, consistency of image quality, and decreased thickness of the imaging slices has rendered CT an important tool in the evaluation of coronary artery disease (CAD). The use of CT for the evaluation of CAD has had volumes written both for and against its use [39, 56–58]. Our brief summarization of these data is that this is a technique greatly overused in young individuals, and likely there is more harm than benefit in much of its use. In older individuals, the risks are less for radiation-induced cancer, and the likelihood of positive results is much greater [59].

There is sufficient evidence on biliary tree imaging evaluation that MRI is clearly superior to CT, and it is also safer than contrast-enhanced cholangiography. MRI, including both tissue imaging contrast-enhanced sequences and MR cholangiopancreatography (MRCP), displays overall topographic display of biliary tree, bile duct wall, and surrounding tissues, and is well accepted by non-imaging physicians because of its depiction of "cholangiographic anatomy" [60–62]. In this clinical setting CT likely plays no substantial role.

Because CT and MRI continue to evolve and improve, it is important to consider the diagnostic accuracy of CT, which is likely to retain advantages over MRI in the foreseeable future. These strengths of CT are based on a few principles: 1) CT is unmatched in its ability to see diseases manifested by the presence of pure calcium or pure air; 2) CT is able to see internal tubes and catheters well; 3) CT is fast; and 4) there is no danger posed to the patient by medical equipment or other objects brought into the scanning room (this is not true of MRI). On the basis of these points, the relative strengths of CT include: examining for renal stones, lung disease especially primary lung disease (such as interstitial lung disease), most acute traumas, and intensive care and other very ill patients in whom the placement of tubes and catheters has to be assessed.

Circumstances in which CT is considered to represent the primary imaging method of evaluation are shown in Table 4.1.

MRI is unlikely to assume a large role in the imaging of many acute severe traumas, owing to the superiority of CT in imaging the full range of lung diseases, and evaluation of the lungs and thorax is often critical in trauma patients. Also a further drawback of MRI in the acute trauma setting is that great care must be taken that no iron-containing metal objects are brought into the scanning room, as these objects can fly into the bore of the magnet, potentially injuring the patient.

Table 4.1 Major clinical indications for CT

Body region	Clinical settings	References
Head	Trauma, brain contusion evaluation, cranial hemorrhage	[63, 64]
Head, mastoid	Trauma, hypoacousia, tumor evaluation, preoperative evaluation for cochlear implant	[65, 66]
Head, paranasal sinuses	Trauma, epistaxis, complicated infection, tumor evaluation	[67, 68]
Spine	Trauma—spinal fracture evaluation	[69, 70]
Chest, lung	Trauma, interstitial lung disease	[71–75]
Chest, wall	Trauma	[73]
Abdomen	Trauma, urolithiasis evaluation	[76–78]
In general	Any region; patients noncooperative and/or in intensive care units	

Serial imaging studies

Distinction should be made between single-use studies (e.g. a serious motor vehicle accident) and serial-use examinations (e.g. follow-up of inflammatory bowel disease such as Crohn's). Single-use studies may not result in unwarranted health risks to the patient when risk–benefit analysis has been performed; however, careful scrutiny should be made of serial-use situations, as consideration must be given to alternative imaging strategies, such as following patients with Crohn's disease, adrenal mass, or complex kidney cysts with MRI. Renal cysts are often sufficiently well evaluated by US, especially in children or thin adults (see below).

What about ultrasound? [79]

Ultrasound (US) is a widely available, noninvasive, innocuous, and safe diagnostic imaging modality; worldwide, it is probably the single most frequently performed exam among all the modern radiologic methods.

Historically, US revolutionized the field of radiology, permitting the first 3D-like visualization of internal organs. From its earliest days to the present, US has played a dominant role in the field of obstetric and reproductive medicine. It remains the most valuable tool for evaluating the normal fetus, and most cases of ovarian morphology and physiology. Many of its other uses vary today because of the concurrent development of both CT and MRI.

To understand which imaging modality should be employed over another, one has to consider the following features: image quality, consistent display of normal and diseased anatomy, availability, cost, patient comfort, and patient safety. These considerations vary at any one time in a given medical center, city, or country.

Major indications for US

The major indications for US comprise: most gynecologic and obstetric evaluations; abdominal illness in children and pregnant patients; all medical situations in which bedside imaging procedure is necessary (acutely ill and trauma patients); intraoperative and interventional imaging guidance; neonatal brain imaging; imaging of superficial structures, such as superficial muscles and tendons (e.g. shoulder rotator cuff), head and neck organs (thyroid, carotid arteries, salivary glands, neck muscles), testicles, prostate, breast masses, and selected vessels (e.g. to evaluate deep vein thrombosis and carotid artery stenosis). Both US and MRI are often used in obstetric and gynecologic settings, in the case of obstetrical cases because of the lack of ionizing radiation. As a rule of thumb, we recommend using US when the disease process is anticipated not to be too complex or malignant, whereas MRI is recommended in complex disease settings and for malignancy.

It is important to distinguish the diagnostic use of US from its use for interventional guidance. Whereas its diagnostic use should be compared with MRI and CT using diagnostic accuracy and safety as measures, its use to guide interventional procedures should be preferred in almost any given situation where the target can be visualized by US, acknowledging its advantages: availability, portability, safety, cost, and flexibility.

The diagnostic use of US worldwide reflects a tremendous variation based on countries' health policies, which ultimately depend on the availability of various machines (US, CT, MR) and experienced physicians in each country. This has impacted directly on the standard of recommended diagnostic strategies, which varies widely among countries. Worldwide, it would appear that countries in which there is availability of modern CT and MRI, the indications of US may be more limited. This therefore would be the case in the USA. Furthermore, US gains in accuracy if the study is performed by physicians experienced in US. Although this is feasible and done in most developing nations, this is generally not performed in developed nations, in part reflecting the time costs of direct physician scanning.

Discussion of specific US indications

Female pelvis and obstetrics

The majority of indications for pelvic US include: 1) pelvic pain, 2) amenorrhea, 3) evaluation of vaginal bleeding (mainly post-menopausal), and 4) palpable mass.

US allows a high confidence of diagnosis of the most common gynecological diseases involving the uterus, fallopian tubes, and ovaries. Higher-resolution imaging is obtained using endovaginal transducers, and this approach has been used as the standard US technique to evaluate the female pelvis over the last decade. High-quality images are generated in a consistent and reproducible manner for localized lesions, although the smaller field of view is a limitation compared with CT and MRI. Hence this is the major reason we advocate MRI for complex or malignant disease.

A great number of female pelvic lesions are detected at sonography, and generally few cases need further imaging evaluation in order to determine an appropriate therapy plan. Although some authors contend that sonography is a reliable method to stage malignancy of the female pelvis, most of these patients are better served with more comprehensive evaluation achievable with MRI [80], as mentioned above. A normal pelvic US exam, in the appropriate clinical setting, carries a high negative predictive value for significant disease processes, which renders US a good screening modality to study the female pelvis [81].

US has been established as the dominant tool for studying normal human development in the first trimester of pregnancy [82]. The advent of high-resolution transvaginal US has revolutionized the understanding of the pathophysiology and the management of early pregnancy failure and is considered the "gold standard" in the diagnosis and management of incomplete miscarriage [82].

Additionally, as radiation exposure should be avoided during pregnancy, US and MRI should be the preferred imaging modalities for evaluating nonobstetrical disease processes of pregnant patients [47, 83]. At our center, complex disease processes such a bowel disease, appendicitis, pancreatitis, and choledocholithiasis are performed with MRI, whereas more localized or superficial processes are investigated by sonography [20, 21, 26, 27].

Pediatric imaging

US is a useful and versatile modality for pediatric imaging, and does not require exposure to radiation or use of sedatives. In many clinical settings, such as the evaluation of abdominal pain, the use of US avoids more costly examinations and the potentially harmful exposure to radiation that CT entails [84]. In this population, the small body *habitus* of children permits the use of high-frequency transducers, which ultimately results in high spatial resolution, improving image consistency and reproducibility.

Acutely ill and trauma patients: Bedside application

Progressively, noninvasive imaging has assumed a prominent role in the evaluation of patients who have acute abdominal conditions. US is often the initial diagnostic imaging modality used to examine patients who are clinically suspected of having acute cholecystitis, and with more variable use in suspected choledocholithiasis and acute appendicitis [85].

Although angiography is the "gold standard" in the evaluation of acute arterial pathologies, Doppler sonography is an accessible, safe, and noninvasive diagnostic modality that may provide prompt and accurate diagnosis concerning an acute emergency of arterial origin [86].

US is being used increasingly in the assessment of acute nontraumatic abdominal pain; however, attention should be paid to the inappropriate use of US by poorly trained users, which can lead to a delayed or incorrect diagnosis, more imaging investigation, and increased hospital costs [87]. As US machines continue to become smaller and more portable, and reduced in cost, more generalized use by nontrained examiners is anticipated. We anticipate that although on the one hand some emergent medical conditions may be detected earlier, on the other hand the expected use by less-well-trained operators likely will result in much greater follow-up use of more expensive modalities, CT and MRI, making health care more expensive, with ultimately more delay, and with possibly more adverse outcomes. We anticipate that future research studies will be published that show widely differing outcomes, invariably influenced by financial incentives.

Breast imaging

US has developed a role in the evaluation of the palpable breast mass, mainly in women younger than 30 years [88, 89]. Although mammography remains the most commonly used modality to screen for breast cancer, a complementary role has been established for US [90]. Because of its intrinsic safety, wider application of sonography, for the evaluation in women younger than 40, would be an important evolution. Recent innovations have suggested that sonography should play a principal role in the evaluation of dense breasts, especially in younger women [91, 92]—a recommendation that we strongly advocate. Recent studies by Weigert et al. [91] and Hooley et al. [92] state that screening breast US in women with dense breasts has a high negative predictive value, sensitivity, and specificity, but low positive predictive value [91]. Both articles report that US screening resulted in an additional 0.8–10 cancers per 1000 women screened with dense breasts [91, 92]. There is no doubt that the future of breast imaging will likely include an increasing role for breast MRI as well [93, 94].

Superficial organs: Testicles, thyroid, carotid, muscle, and tendons

US is the initial imaging performed in patients with acute scrotum, and its ability to diagnose the pathogenesis of acute scrotum is unsurpassed by any other imaging modality [95]. It is the fastest approach to assess testicular vasculature to evaluate for torsion. The high-resolution images obtained with high-frequency linear transducers can demonstrate extra- and intratesticular pathology in detail [96, 97]. MRI has been used to evaluate unsolved cases of scrotal pathology [98].

US is the best imaging modality available to evaluate thyroid nodules, to a great extent reflecting the superficial location of this organ. US findings on their own often determine the clinical management of the majority of patients referred after abnormal results on thyroid physical examination [99]. Specificity of US findings alone is not sufficiently high to diagnose cancer; thus many patients will require fine-needle aspiration, which may be performed at the same time using US guidance [100]. Our impression is that one area of considerable overuse of imaging—biopsy and histopatho-logic evaluation—is in the evaluation of the thyroid gland. Clearly further research is needed to more accurately triage patients into whether they need US and/or biopsy. This is currently beyond the scope of this book.

Noninvasive screening for carotid artery stenosis has been most often performed by US and MRI. Many studies have described the superiority of MRI in the detection of significant carotid stenosis; nonetheless, many groups have used US alone in select patients as preoperative evaluation prior to carotid endarterectomy [101, 102].

Musculoskeletal US has become a well-established diagnostic method in recent years [103]. US can diagnose tears of muscles and tendons, tendi-nosis, and tenosynovitis in superficial locations [104]. Dynamic assessment of joints can also be performed with sonography. Apart from plain film evaluation for trauma and as a first-line tool to assess possible bone tumors, MRI is the primary diagnostic tool in the evaluation of muscu-loskeletal disease because of the detailed diagnostic information provided [105]. MRI is often critical for the staging of tumors of the musculoskeletal system. The technique also has widespread utility in the evaluation of connective tissue and anatomy of the knee, hip joint, shoulder, and other structures [105]. The complementary use of US and MRI in selected cases has been found to be advantageous [106].

Gallbladder and biliary tree evaluation

US is often employed as the initial imaging modality for the evaluation of suspected acute gallbladder disorders, and is often sufficient for correct diagnosis [107].

Biliary tree evaluation has been a common indication for US, with one report describing US as accurate for virtually all cases of intrahepatic biliary dilatation [108]. However, in our experience, and that of most centers, common bile duct evaluation by US has variable and most often insuffi-cient success, reflecting many factors such as: operator experience, patient's body *habitus,* complexity of disease, and quality of machinery. In most settings MRI should be used to evaluate the common bile duct, as it is the most successful at detecting choledocholithiasis, and detecting and staging various cancers.

Screening of hepatocellular carcinoma

Abdominal US is widely used as a screening tool for hepatocellular carcinoma (HCC) in cirrhotic patients, although US is generally performed for this indication in developing countries. In our experience, many HCCs can be missed with sonography, and MRI should be routinely used in all these patients in developed nations. Nonetheless, it should be acknowledged that recent studies generally indicate a 60% sensitivity or higher, a specificity greater than 90%, and a positive predictive value of 70% [109–113], although we consider these numbers insufficient for its use. One study performed by Lin et al., comparing US, CT, and alpha-fetoprotein strategies, concluded that biannual alpha-fetoprotein/annual US gives the most quality-adjusted life-year gain while still maintaining a cost-effectiveness ratio <$50.000/quality-adjusted life-year [114]. This approach is recommended by other authors [115–117]. A recent meta-analysis, by Yuen and Lai [118], considered that both US and alpha-fetoprotein testing have a low sensitivity for detecting HCC, although their combination can increase sensitivity. Even so, both examinations remain the main screening methods for HCC worldwide because they are convenient, noninvasive, and easily available [118]. Nonetheless, Sherman [119] considered that the major drawback to using US for HCC screening is that it is very operator-dependent—because of that, ideally sonographers performing HCC screening should receive special training, much as it is done for mammographic screening in some jurisdictions [119]. In the end, it is our experience that the best imaging modality to evaluate for HCC is MRI with gadolinium enhancement.

Renal and prostate evaluation

US is commonly used to evaluate the kidneys and the urinary tract. There are specific indications, most related to the urinary tract evaluation of children and pregnant women [120]. Many of these indications are to evaluate acute-onset flank pain, suspected stone disease, hematuria, and renal failure. Nonetheless, because of the limited ability of US to demonstrate kidney physiology (e.g. enhancement properties), CT and MRI play the major role in kidney evaluation.

To date, nonenhanced CT is the best modality to assess urinary tract stone disease [121]. US has a role following up renal cystic masses that have been characterized by CT or MRI [122]. Incidental renal cancers can be discovered by US, but CT or MRI must be utilized to stage renal malignancy [123].

US has become an essential component of the management of renal transplantation [124]. Because of the superficial location of the transplanted kidney, US is the most widely used imaging modality to follow up the transplanted allograft to detect suspected complications. Doppler US has been particularly important for studying vascular compromise.

Doppler US can be used to screen patients for renovascular hypertension, but CT and MRI are significantly more accurate for the diagnosis of atherosclerotic renal artery stenosis [125]. In our experience, MRI should be preferred for kidneys and urinary tract evaluation, with the exception of stone disease, which is better studied by nonenhanced CT. The major problem with CT in this clinical setting, however, is its tremendous overuse [31].

Transrectal US (TRUS) is a useful method for assessing prostate pathology, and it plays an important role for prostate cancer screening in concert with prostate-specific antigen and digital rectal examination [126]. Despite the technological advances of TRUS for the detection of prostate cancer, such as color and power Doppler US, harmonic imaging and contrast-enhanced US techniques, US accuracy for cancer diagnosis cannot preclude TRUS-guided systematic core biopsy of the prostate at the present time [127]. MRI and MR spectroscopy may become the most sensitive tools for the noninvasive, anatomic, and metabolic evaluation of prostate cancer [128, 129].

TRUS has a major role in the evaluation of male infertility looking for abnormalities in the ejaculatory ducts, seminal vesicles, and vas deferens [130].

Drawbacks of US

US examination is a highly operator-dependent procedure. All findings must be identified during the scanning procedure. If some region is not scanned, or, if it is scanned but the disease was not perceived at time of scanning, it is very unlikely that findings will be identified at the time of image interpretation. There are new attempts to solve this problem using digitally recording apparatus, most often using 3D US data, but recording large examinations leads to a long review process. Because of that, sonographers and radiologists must be adept at *"fast" or "real-time"* anatomy–pathology correlation. Often interaction with the patient provides clinical information that aids clarification of imaging findings. The advantages of CT and MRI examinations is that they can be read and reviewed more than once by the primary reviewer, or by secondary readers, due to their intrinsic overall topographic display, which generally is not performed or achievable with US.

Another drawback is that US is more time-consuming than CT or MRI. This is especially true when radiologists are performing the scanning themselves. During the time that one US exam is performed by one experienced radiologist, three or more CT or MRI exams could be interpreted. A study addressing the cost-effectiveness of obstetric US considered that the sonographers' skills in detecting anomalies and the time taken to perform a scan have a significant effect on the relative cost-effectiveness of the method [131].

The patient's body *habitus* also has a major effect on US—more so than with CT and MRI. Suboptimal body *habitus*, usually reflecting obesity, results in reduction of the penetration of the sound waves within the body, restricting field of view and spatial resolution. Fatty tissue and air, in structures such as bowel, are major limitations to image quality and diagnostic accuracy of US. It must be recalled that obesity is a common affliction in the North American population, so this limitation is frequently encountered. Improvements during the last decade of US technology, such as the implementation of harmonic imaging, have diminished this problem.

Acceptance of US examinations, especially by surgeons, is often low because of lack of an easily recognizable display of anatomy. CT and MRI provide images of greater topographic anatomical display. MRCP is an example of a technique with high physician acceptance.

Ideal solution

The ideal circumstance is that constant reevaluation is performed among imaging modalities evaluating comparative effectiveness. When safer modalities show superior or comparable results for a particular clinical setting they should be used extensively, or even exclusively, in that setting. Concurrent evolution of CT into the use of lower amounts of radiation exposure should also be factored into safety considerations on the plus side of CT. We have adopted a threshold of 1 mSv as the level to carefully scrutinize the use of an ionizing-energy-based imaging modality [132]. So on the newest CT scanners and newest reconstruction methods, CT use may again be advocated if the radiation exposure drops below this. As mentioned in earlier chapters, the initial critical determination is whether any imaging study should be performed at all, as a starting point.

Workable solution

Specific clinical settings

Summarizing information from above, there is no group in which substitution of ionizing-radiation-based imaging by non-ionizing-radiation-based imaging is more imperative than in the pediatric population. Following several high-profile cases in which children were overexposed to medical radiation, a workshop organized by the Food and Drug Administration (FDA) mandated improvements in medical devices for pediatric imaging [133]. For this reason we emphasize the need to substitute either MRI or US for CT in pediatric and young adult settings, not only when they are better or equivalent, but also where CT may be a little better. An example of this is the evaluation for acute appendicitis.

References

1. Nelson HD, Tyne K, Naik A, et al. Screening for breast cancer: An update for the U.S. Preventive Services Task Force. Ann Intern Med 2009; 151:727–737, W237–742.
2. Woloshin S, Schwartz LM. How a charity oversells mammography. BMJ 2012; 345:e5132.
3. Reynolds H. When a mammogram is riskier than cancer. Bloomberg 2012. Available online at: http://www.bloomberg.com/news/2012-08-02/when-a-mammogram-is-riskier-than-cancer.html [accessed February 27, 2013].
4. Davisson L. Rational care or rationing care? Updates and controversies in women's prevention. W V Med J 2012; 108:70–76.
5. Gold LS, Klein G, Carr L, et al. The emergence of diagnostic imaging technologies in breast cancer: Discovery, regulatory approval, reimbursement, and adoption in clinical guidelines. Cancer Imaging 2012; 12:13–24.
6. Lannin DR. Realistic appraisal of the benefits of mammography. Arch Intern Med 2012; 172:672–673.
7. Looking back on the millennium in medicine. N Eng J Med 2000; 342:42–49.
8. Flynn K. Assessing diagnostic technologies. In: Technology Assessment Program. Report No. 1. Boston, MA: Veterans Health Administration's Office of Research and Development, 1996; 1–15.

9. Bossuyt PM, Reitsma JB, Bruns DE, et al. Towards complete and accurate reporting of studies of diagnostic accuracy: The STARD initiative. Bmj 2003; 326:41–44.

10. Bossuyt PM, Reitsma JB, Bruns DE, et al. Towards complete and accurate reporting of studies of diagnostic accuracy: The STARD Initiative. Ann Intern Med 2003; 138:40–44.

11. Moher D, Schulz KF, Altman DG. The CONSORT statement: Revised recommendations for improving the quality of reports of parallel-group randomised trials. Lancet 2001; 357:1191–1194.

12. Fryback DG, Thornbury JR. The efficacy of diagnostic imaging. Med Decis Making 1991; 11:88–94.

13. Burgess CA, Dale OT, Almeyda R, et al. An evidence based review of the assessment and management of penetrating neck trauma. Clin Otolaryngol 2012; 37:44–52.

14. Osmond MH, Klassen TP, Wells GA, et al. CATCH: A clinical decision rule for the use of computed tomography in children with minor head injury. CMAJ 2010; 182:341–348.

15. Rhea JT, Garza DH, Novelline RA. Controversies in emergency radiology. CT versus ultrasound in the evaluation of blunt abdominal trauma. Emerg Radiol 2004; 10:289–295.

16. Shiga T, Wajima Z, Apfel CC, et al. Diagnostic accuracy of transesophageal echocardiography, helical computed tomography, and magnetic resonance imaging for suspected thoracic aortic dissection: Systematic review and meta-analysis. Arch Intern Med 2006; 166:1350–1356.

17. Hayter RG, Rhea JT, Small A, et al. Suspected aortic dissection and other aortic disorders: Multi-detector row CT in 373 cases in the emergency setting. Radiology 2006; 238:841–852.

18. Yoshida S, Akiba H, Tamakawa M, et al. Thoracic involvement of type A aortic dissection and intramural hematoma: Diagnostic accuracy-comparison of emergency helical CT and surgical findings. Radiology 2003; 228:430–435.

19. Hong JJ, Cohn SM, Ekeh AP, et al. A prospective randomized study of clinical assessment versus computed tomography for the diagnosis of acute appendicitis. Surg Infect (Larchmt) 2003; 4:231–239.

20. Birchard KR, Brown MA, Hyslop WB, et al. MRI of acute abdominal and pelvic pain in pregnant patients. AJR Am J Roentgenol 2005; 184:452–458.

21. Oto A, Ernst RD, Ghulmiyyah LM, et al. MR imaging in the triage of pregnant patients with acute abdominal and pelvic pain. Abdom Imaging 2009; 34: 243–250.

22. Pedrosa I, Lafornara M, Pandharipande PV, et al. Pregnant patients suspected of having acute appendicitis: effect of MR imaging on negative laparotomy rate and appendiceal perforation rate. Radiology 2009; 250:749–757.

23. Markar SR, Karthikesalingam A, Cunningham J, et al. Increased use of preoperative imaging and laparoscopy has no impact on clinical outcomes in patients undergoing appendicectomy. Ann R Coll Surg Engl 2011; 93:620–623.

24. Pritchett CV, Levinsky NC, Ha YP, et al. Management of acute appendicitis: The impact of CT scanning on the bottom line. J Am Coll Surg 2010; 210:699–705, 705–697.

25. Krajewski S, Brown J, Phang PT, et al. Impact of computed tomography of the abdomen on clinical outcomes in patients with acute right lower quadrant pain: A meta-analysis. Can J Surg 2011; 54:43–53.

26. Brown MA, Birchard KR, Semelka RC. Magnetic resonance evaluation of pregnant patients with acute abdominal pain. Semin Ultrasound CT MR 2005; 26: 206–211.

27. Oto A, Ernst RD, Shah R, et al. Right-lower-quadrant pain and suspected appendicitis in pregnant women: evaluation with MR imaging-initial experience. Radiology 2005; 234:445–451.

28. Niemann T, Kollmann T, Bongartz G. Diagnostic performance of low-dose CT for the detection of urolithiasis: A meta-analysis. AJR Am J Roentgenol 2008; 191:396–401.

29. Shine S. Urinary calculus: IVU vs. CT renal stone? A critically appraised topic. Abdom Imaging 2008; 33:41–43.

30. Worster A, Preyra I, Weaver B, et al. The accuracy of noncontrast helical computed tomography versus intravenous pyelography in the diagnosis of suspected acute urolithiasis: A meta-analysis. Ann Emerg Med 2002; 40:280–286.

31. Poletti PA, Platon A, Rutschmann OT, et al. Abdominal plain film in patients admitted with clinical suspicion of renal colic: Should it be replaced by low-dose computed tomography? Urology 2006; 67:64–68.

32. Stein PD, Woodard PK, Weg JG, et al. Diagnostic pathways in acute pulmonary embolism: Recommendations of the PIOPED II investigators. Am J Med 2006; 119:1048–1055.

33. Schoepf UJ, Helmberger T, Holzknecht N, et al. Segmental and subsegmental pulmonary arteries: Evaluation with electron-beam versus spiral CT. Radiology 2000; 214:433–439.

34. Heredia V, Ramalho M, Zapparoli M, et al. Incidence of pulmonary embolism and other chest findings in younger patients using multidetector computed tomography. Acta Radiol 2010; 51:402–406.

35. Burns SK, Haramati LB. Diagnostic imaging and risk stratification of patients with acute pulmonary embolism. Cardiol Rev 2012; 20:15–24.

36. Altun E, Heredia V, Pamuklar E, et al. Feasibility of post-gadolinium three-dimensional gradient-echo sequence to evaluate the pulmonary arterial vasculature. Magn Reson Imaging 2009; 27:1198–1207.

37. Santos MK, Elias J, Jr., Mauad FM, et al. Magnetic resonance imaging of the chest: Current and new applications, with an emphasis on pulmonology. J Bras Pneumol 2011; 37:242–258.

38. Altun E, Elias J, Jr, Birchard KR, et al. Chest. In: Semelka RC, ed. Abdominal-pelvic MRI. 3rd edn. Hoboken, New Jersey: John Wiley & Sons, 2010; 1653–1686.

39. Hoffmann U, Truong QA, Schoenfeld DA, et al. Coronary CT angiography versus standard evaluation in acute chest pain. N Engl J Med 2012; 367:299–308.

40. Martin DR, Semelka RC. Health effects of ionising radiation from diagnostic CT. Lancet 2006; 367:1712–1714.

41. Semelka RC. Abdominal-pelvic MRI. Hoboken, New Jersey: John Wiley & Sons, 2010.

42. Lauenstein TC, Goehde SC, Herborn CU, et al. Whole-body MR imaging: Evaluation of patients for metastases. Radiology 2004; 233:139–148.

43. Bulas D, Goske M, Applegate K, et al. Image Gently: Improving health literacy for parents about CT scans for children. Pediatr Radiol 2009; 39:112–116.

44. Goske MJ, Applegate KE, Boylan J, et al. The Image Gently campaign: Working together to change practice. AJR Am J Roentgenol 2008; 190:273–274.

45. Goske MJ, Applegate KE, Boylan J, et al. The 'Image Gently' campaign: increasing CT radiation dose awareness through a national education and awareness program. Pediatr Radiol 2008; 38:265–269.

46. Semelka RC, Martin DR, Balci C, et al. Focal liver lesions: Comparison of dual-phase CT and multisequence multiplanar MR imaging including dynamic gadolinium enhancement. J Magn Reson Imaging 2001; 13:397–401.

47. Birchard KR, Semelka RC, Hyslop WB, et al. Suspected pancreatic cancer: Evaluation by dynamic gadolinium-enhanced 3D gradient-echo MRI. AJR Am J Roentgenol 2005; 185:700–703.

48. Pamuklar E, Semelka RC. MR imaging of the pancreas. Magn Reson Imaging Clin N Am 2005; 13:313–330.

49. Noone TC, Hosey J, Firat Z, et al. Imaging and localization of islet-cell tumours of the pancreas on CT and MRI. Best Pract Res Clin Endocrinol Metab 2005; 19:195–211.

50. Kim JK, Altun E, Elias J, Jr., et al. Focal pancreatic mass: Distinction of pancreatic cancer from chronic pancreatitis using gadolinium-enhanced 3D-gradient-echo MRI. J Magn Reson Imaging 2007; 26:313–322.

51. Balci NC, Semelka RC. Radiologic diagnosis and staging of pancreatic ductal adenocarcinoma. Eur J Radiol 2001; 38:105–112.

52. Elias J, Jr., Semelka RC, Altun E, et al. Pancreatic cancer: Correlation of MR findings, clinical features, and tumor grade. J Magn Reson Imaging 2007; 26: 1556–1563.

53. Shin SS, Armao DM, Burke LM, et al. Comparison of the incidence of pancreatic abnormalities between high risk and control patients: Prospective pilot study with 3 Tesla MR imaging. J Magn Reson Imaging 2011; 33:1080–1085.

54. Kelekis NL, Semelka RC, Molina PL, et al. ACTH-secreting islet cell tumor: appearances on dynamic gadolinium-enhanced MRI. Magn Reson Imaging 1995; 13:641–644.

55. Semelka RC, Cumming MJ, Shoenut JP, et al. Islet cell tumors: Comparison of dynamic contrast-enhanced CT and MR imaging with dynamic gadolinium enhancement and fat suppression. Radiology 1993; 186:799–802.

56. Litt HI, Gatsonis C, Snyder B, et al. CT angiography for safe discharge of patients with possible acute coronary syndromes. N Engl J Med 2012; 366:1393–1403.

57. Min JK, Kang N, Shaw LJ, et al. Costs and clinical outcomes after coronary multidetector CT angiography in patients without known coronary artery disease: Comparison to myocardial perfusion SPECT. Radiology 2008; 249:62–70.

58. Takakuwa KM, Keith SW, Estepa AT, et al. A meta-analysis of 64-section coronary CT angiography findings for predicting 30-day major adverse cardiac events in patients presenting with symptoms suggestive of acute coronary syndrome. Acad Radiol 2011; 18:1522–1528.

59. Blankstein R, Ahmed W, Bamberg F, et al. Comparison of exercise treadmill testing with cardiac computed tomography angiography among patients presenting to the emergency room with chest pain: The Rule Out Myocardial Infarction Using

Computer-Assisted Tomography (ROMICAT) study. Circ Cardiovasc Imaging 2012; 5:233–242.

60. Ferrari FS, Fantozzi F, Tasciotti L, et al. US, MRCP, CCT and ERCP: A comparative study in 131 patients with suspected biliary obstruction. Med Sci Monit 2005; 11:MT8–18.
61. Hyodo T, Kumano S, Kushihata F, et al. CT and MR cholangiography: Advantages and pitfalls in perioperative evaluation of biliary tree. Br J Radiol 2012; 85:887–896.
62. Dave M, Elmunzer BJ, Dwamena BA, eta l. Primary sclerosing cholangitis: Meta-analysis of diagnostic performance of MR cholangiopancreatography. Radiology 2010; 256:387–396.
63. Davis PC, Wippold II FJ, Cornelius RS, et al. Head trauma. ACR Appropriateness Criteria® 2012. Available online at: http://www.acr.org/~/media/ACR/Documents/AppCriteria/Diagnostic/HeadTrauma.pdf. [accessed February 27, 2013].
64. Masdeu JC, Irimia P, Asenbaum S, et al. EFNS guideline on neuroimaging in acute stroke. Report of an EFNS task force. Eur J Neurol 2006; 13:1271–1283.
65. St Martin MB, Hirsch BE. Imaging of hearing loss. Otolaryngol Clin North Am 2008; 41:157–178, vi–vii.
66. Cerini R, Faccioli N, Cicconi D, et al. Role of CT and MRI in the preoperative evaluation of auditory brainstem implantation in patients with congenital inner ear pathology. Radiol Med 2006; 111:978–988.
67. Madani G, Beale TJ, Lund VJ. Imaging of sinonasal tumors. Semin Ultrasound CT MR 2009; 30:25–38.
68. Wippold FJ, 2nd. Head and neck imaging: The role of CT and MRI. J Magn Reson Imaging 2007; 25:453–465.
69. Bagley LJ. Imaging of spinal trauma. Radiol Clin North Am 2006; 44:1–12, vii.
70. Gonzalez-Beicos A, Nunez DB, Jr. Role of multidetector computed tomography in the assessment of cervical spine trauma. Semin Ultrasound CT MR 2009; 30:159–167.
71. Caterino U. Computed tomography changing over time in type 1 pulmonary laceration. Ann Emerg Med 2009; 54:156–157.
72. Kaewlai R, Avery LL, Asrani AV, et al. Multidetector CT of blunt thoracic trauma. Radiographics 2008; 28:1555–1570.
73. Magu S, Yadav A, Agarwal S. Computed tomography in blunt chest trauma. Indian J Chest Dis Allied Sci 2009; 51:75–81.
74. Argiriadi PA, Mendelson DS. High resolution computed tomography in idiopathic interstitial pneumonias. Mt Sinai J Med 2009; 76:37–52.
75. Sung A, Swigris J, Saleh A, et al. High-resolution chest tomography in idiopathic pulmonary fibrosis and nonspecific interstitial pneumonia: Utility and challenges. Curr Opin Pulm Med 2007; 13:451–457.
76. Hamidi MI, Aldaoud KM, Qtaish I. The role of computed tomography in blunt abdominal trauma. Sultan Qaboos Univ Med J 2007; 7:41–46.
77. Stuhlfaut JW, Anderson SW, Soto JA. Blunt abdominal trauma: Current imaging techniques and CT findings in patients with solid organ, bowel, and mesenteric injury. Semin Ultrasound CT MR 2007; 28:115–129.
78. Silverman SG, Leyendecker JR, Amis ES, Jr. What is the current role of CT urography and MR urography in the evaluation of the urinary tract? Radiology 2009; 250:309–323.

79. Elias J, Jr., Semelka RC. Utility of ultrasound in the modern imaging paradigm. Medscape Radiology Education 2006. Available online at: http://www.medscape.com/viewprogram/6094_pnt [accessed March 5, 2013].

80. Devine C, Szklaruk J, Tamm EP. Magnetic resonance imaging in the characterization of pelvic masses. Semin Ultrasound CT MR 2005; 26:172–204.

81. Okaro E, Valentin L. The role of ultrasound in the management of women with acute and chronic pelvic pain. Best Pract Res Clin Obstet Gynaecol 2004; 18:105–123.

82. Jauniaux E, Johns J, Burton GJ. The role of ultrasound imaging in diagnosing and investigating early pregnancy failure. Ultrasound Obstet Gynecol 2005; 25:613–624.

83. Bau A, Atri M. Acute female pelvic pain: Ultrasound evaluation. Semin Ultrasound CT MR 2000; 21:78–93.

84. Schmidt RE, Babcock DS, Farrell MK. Use of abdominal and pelvic ultrasound in the evaluation of chronic abdominal pain. Clin Pediatr (Phila) 1993; 32: 147–150.

85. Laing FC. Ultrasonography of the acute abdomen. Radiol Clin North Am 1992; 30:389–404.

86. Kantarci F, Mihmanli I, Kara B, et al. Acute arterial emergencies: Evaluation by Doppler ultrasound. Emerg Radiol 2005; 11:315–321.

87. Raman S, Somasekar K, Winter RK, et al. Are we overusing ultrasound in non-traumatic acute abdominal pain? Postgrad Med J 2004; 80:177–179.

88. Buchberger W, Niehoff A, Obrist P, et al. Clinically and mammographically occult breast lesions: Detection and classification with high-resolution sonography. Semin Ultrasound CT MR 2000; 21:325–336.

89. Zonderland HM. The role of ultrasound in the diagnosis of breast cancer. Semin Ultrasound CT MR 2000; 21:317–324.

90. Elmore JG, Armstrong K, Lehman CD, et al. Screening for breast cancer. JAMA 2005; 293:1245–1256.

91. Weigert J, Steenbergen S. The connecticut experiment: The role of ultrasound in the screening of women with dense breasts. Breast J 2012; 18:517–522.

92. Hooley RJ, Greenberg KL, Stackhouse RM, et al. Screening US in patients with mammographically dense breasts: Initial experience with Connecticut Public Act 09–41. Radiology 2012; 265:59–69.

93. Ikeda DM, Baker DR, Daniel BL. Magnetic resonance imaging of breast cancer: Clinical indications and breast MRI reporting system. J Magn Reson Imaging 2000; 12:975–983.

94. Bartella L, Morris EA. Advances in breast imaging: Magnetic resonance imaging. Curr Oncol Rep 2006; 8:7–13.

95. Dogra V, Bhatt S. Acute painful scrotum. Radiol Clin North Am 2004; 42: 349–363.

96. Oyen RH. Scrotal ultrasound. Eur Radiol 2002; 12:19–34.

97. Blaivas M, Brannam L. Testicular ultrasound. Emerg Med Clin North Am 2004; 22:723–748, ix.

98. Muglia V, Tucci S, Jr., Elias J, Jr., et al. Magnetic resonance imaging of scrotal diseases: when it makes the difference. Urology 2002; 59:419–423.

99. Marqusee E, Benson CB, Frates MC, et al. Usefulness of ultrasonography in the management of nodular thyroid disease. Ann Intern Med 2000; 133:696–700.

100. Frates MC, Benson CB, Charboneau JW, et al. Management of thyroid nodules detected at US: Society of Radiologists in Ultrasound consensus conference statement. Radiology 2005; 237:794–800.

101. Nederkoorn PJ, Mali WP, Eikelboom BC, et al. Preoperative diagnosis of carotid artery stenosis: Accuracy of noninvasive testing. Stroke 2002; 33:2003–2008.

102. Engelhardt M, Bruijnen H, Schnur C, et al. Duplex scanning criteria for selection of patients for internal carotid artery endarterectomy. Vasa 2005; 34:36–40.

103. Martinoli C, Bianchi S, Dahmane M, et al. Ultrasound of tendons and nerves. Eur Radiol 2002; 12:44–55.

104. Torriani M, Kattapuram SV. Musculoskeletal ultrasound: An alternative imaging modality for sports-related injuries. Top Magn Reson Imaging 2003; 14:103–111.

105. Bluemke D. Musculoskeletal MRI: New Imaging Strategies Emerge. In: Medscape, 2001.

106. Adler RS, Finzel KC. The complementary roles of MR imaging and ultrasound of tendons. Radiol Clin North Am 2005; 43:771–807, ix.

107. Bennett GL, Balthazar EJ. Ultrasound and CT evaluation of emergent gallbladder pathology. Radiol Clin North Am 2003; 41:1203–1216.

108. Yarmenitis SD. Ultrasound of the gallbladder and the biliary tree. Eur Radiol 2002; 12:270–282.

109. Takayasu K, Moriyama N, Muramatsu Y, et al. The diagnosis of small hepatocellular carcinomas: Efficacy of various imaging procedures in 100 patients. AJR Am J Roentgenol 1990; 155:49–54.

110. Solmi L, Primerano AM, Gandolfi L. Ultrasound follow-up of patients at risk for hepatocellular carcinoma: Results of a prospective study on 360 cases. Am J Gastroenterol 1996; 91:1189–1194.

111. Larcos G, Sorokopud H, Berry G, et al. Sonographic screening for hepatocellular carcinoma in patients with chronic hepatitis or cirrhosis: An evaluation. AJR Am J Roentgenol 1998; 171:433–435.

112. Chen TH, Chen CJ, Yen MF, et al. Ultrasound screening and risk factors for death from hepatocellular carcinoma in a high risk group in Taiwan. Int J Cancer 2002; 98:257–261.

113. Pateron D, Ganne N, Trinchet JC, et al. Prospective study of screening for hepatocellular carcinoma in Caucasian patients with cirrhosis. J Hepatol 1994; 20: 65–71.

114. Lin OS, Keeffe EB, Sanders GD, Owns DK. Cost-effectiveness of screening for hepatocellular carcinoma in patients with cirrhosis due to chronic hepatitis C. Aliment Pharmacol Ther 2004; 19:1159–1172.

115. Ruelas-Villavicencio AL, Vargas-Vorackova F. In whom, how and how often is surveillance for hepatocellular carcinoma cost-effective? Ann Hepatol 2004; 3:152–159.

116. Patel D, Terrault NA, Yao FY, Bass NM, Ladabaum U. Cost-effectiveness of hepatocellular carcinoma surveillance in patients with hepatitis C virus-related cirrhosis. Clin Gastroenterol Hepatol 2005; 3:75–84.

117. Daniele B, Bencivenga A, Megna AS, et al. Alpha-fetoprotein and ultrasonography screening for hepatocellular carcinoma. Gastroenterology 2004; 127:S108–112.

118. Yuen MF, Lai CL. Screening for hepatocellular carcinoma: Survival benefit and cost-effectiveness. Ann Oncol 2003; 14:1463–1467.

119. Sherman M. Screening for hepatocellular carcinoma. Best Pract Res Clin Gastro-enterol 2005; 19:101–118.

120. Noble VE, Brown DF. Renal ultrasound. Emerg Med Clin North Am 2004; 22:641–659.

121. Rao PN. Imaging for kidney stones. World J Urol 2004; 22:323–327.

122. Hartman DS, Choyke PL, Hartman MS. From the RSNA refresher courses: A practical approach to the cystic renal mass. Radiographics 2004; 24 Suppl 1:S101–115.

123. Helenon O, Correas JM, Balleyguier C, et al. Ultrasound of renal tumors. Eur Radiol 2001; 11:1890–1901.

124. de Morais RH, Muglia VF, Mamere AE, et al. Duplex Doppler sonography of transplant renal artery stenosis. J Clin Ultrasound 2003; 31:135–141.

125. Leiner T, de Haan MW, Nelemans PJ, et al. Contemporary imaging techniques for the diagnosis of renal artery stenosis. Eur Radiol 2005; 15:2219–2229.

126. Clements R. Ultrasonography of prostate cancer. Eur Radiol 2001; 11: 2119–2125.

127. Ismail M, Gomella LG. Ultrasound for prostate imaging and biopsy. Curr Opin Urol 2001; 11:471–477.

128. Hricak H. MR imaging and MR spectroscopic imaging in the pre-treatment evaluation of prostate cancer. Br J Radiol 2005; 78 Spec No 2:S103–111.

129. Rajesh A, Coakley FV. MR imaging and MR spectroscopic imaging of prostate cancer. Magn Reson Imaging Clin N Am 2004; 12:557–579, vii.

130. Zahalsky M, Nagler HM. Ultrasound and infertility: Diagnostic and therapeutic uses. Curr Urol Rep 2001; 2:437–442.

131. Bricker L, Garcia J, Henderson J, et al. Ultrasound screening in pregnancy: A systematic review of the clinical effectiveness, cost-effectiveness and women's views. Health Technol Assess 2000; 4:i–vi, 1–193.

132. Semelka RC, Armao DM, Elias J, Jr., et al. The information imperative: Is it time for an informed consent process explaining the risks of medical radiation? Radiology 2012; 262:15–18.

133. Keen C. FDA workshop explores pediatric radiation dose. Available online at: http://www.drbicuspid.com/index.aspx?Sec=sup&sub=img&pag=dis&ItemID=311019&wf=47 [accessed February 27, 2013].

CHAPTER 5

Patient information

Jorge Elias Jr[1] and Richard C. Semelka[2]
[1] The School of Medicine of Ribeirao Preto, University of Sao Paulo, Brazil
[2] University of North Carolina at Chapel Hill, School of Medicine, Department of Radiology, Chapel Hill, NC, USA

In all of medicine there are a variety of strategies that can be used to diagnose or treat patients, with relatively sparse real-life comparative effectiveness data. Under this uncertainty, traditionally physicians have advised the patient on what they consider the best approach, in essence purportedly acting as their fiduciary. Unfortunately, however, all individuals, including physicians, have bias: and generally that bias leans toward procedures that the particular physician is somehow beneficiary of. This circumstance may largely remain insolvable. What should be clear, however, is that in all medical procedures that involve some level of risk, patients should be made aware of these risks, so that they can determine a risk–benefit evaluation that is acceptable to them. Recently this approach of incorporating the patient into their health care decision making, part of the concept of patient-centered medicine, has received the moniker "shared decision making." This current approach is gaining traction in medical care as an appropriate means to manage patients. Through this process, patients and providers consider outcome probabilities and patient preferences and reach a health care decision based on mutual agreement. Although shared decision making has established a presence in clinical medicine, we will introduce this concept for Radiology. The foundation, though, is providing patients with access to information on procedures that they are recommended to undergo—what we have termed the Information Imperative.

Scope of the issue

Providing information to patients about their disease processes and the intended medical procedures to remedy them is an essential part of the physician–patient relationship. This forms the basis of the discussion with patients on risk–benefit analysis of their case [1]. Doctor–patient relationship can be classified in four basic forms: default, paternalistic, consumerist, and mutualistic [2]. Default relationships are characterized by a lack of control on either side, and hence are generally far from ideal. Paternalism is characterized by the dominant role of the doctor dictating care and the passive role of patients accepting that care. This form of physician–patient relationship has dominated health care largely from its inception to the 1980s. Consumerism is a recent approach, since the 1980s, facilitated by widely available information of all levels of credibility on the Internet, where the focus is on patients' rights and doctors' obligations. Mutuality is characterized by a sharing of decision making, which clearly is the most balanced approach, and in the current times often advocated as the best type of patient–physician relationship. This is currently now described as shared decision-making.

The case of informed consent for medical radiation

As it is beyond question that ionizing radiation, arguably when it may reach a certain exposure level, poses health risks to exposed individuals, the most important of which is cancer induction, it would seem reasonable that information about these risks be conveyed to patients. Information delivery may be conveyed by passive or active means. "Passive information delivery" reflects the fact that information is provided based on the initiative of the patients—either by their request of the health care workers servicing them, or by their efforts to search out this information, often using the Internet as the source. It would appear that radiology departments at present generally provide information to patients when the patients themselves initiate that request.

It is our contention that risks of medical radiation should be conveyed in an active manner. There are three common methods of active health care information delivery to patients: 1) provision of written material; 2) verbal communication (verbal informed consent); and 3) verbal communication documented in writing with consent affirmed with the subject's signature (written informed consent). At the present time none of these forms of active communication about the health risks of exposure to ionizing radiation during medical imaging procedures are in common use, and our opinion is that it behooves imaging specialists to be more forthcoming to inform patients of potential risks associated with imaging examinations.

The informed consent process in the USA arose from two court decisions in the early 1970s—one in California [3], one in Washington, DC [4]—that held that there is a duty owed to patients by health care providers to obtain their informed consent, explaining risks, benefits, and alternative treatments. The failure to obtain the informed consent from a patient appropriately is medical malpractice. The administration of informed consent regulations is a state issue and not a federal law issue, which renders generalizing a strategy across the USA somewhat problematic. Wide variation exists in the requirements among individual states for documentation of the informed consent process [5]. In fact, many states, such as North Carolina, do not require written documentation of informed consent.

The concept of informed consent refers to the actual discussion between health care provider and patient. This process should provide sufficiently complete information to allow the patient to understand the implications of the decision, to make their informed decision, and to communicate their decision to the health care provider. The value of memorializing this consent process in writing is that there is a legal presumption that consent was properly obtained if there is a written and signed consent form. It is easier to prove that informed consent was obtained if there is a signed document. This practice has been adopted worldwide [6–8]. Generally, obtaining written informed consent has been in general practice for all "invasive" radiological procedures—that is, for procedures that enter the physical domain of the patient. The most common reason for obtaining written informed consent in Radiology is for the range of interventional radiology procedures that are imaging-based and involve inserting devices into the patient.

The discussion of risks of general medical procedures with patients has generally focused on iatrogenic misadventures that occur in the acute phase after the procedure (i.e. within 48 hours). The need for informed consent (whether verbal or written) when the bodily integrity of the patient has not been encroached upon or when the adverse event may arise in the chronic phase (i.e. more than 1 month post-procedure) has been considered [9], but no governing body in the USA has enacted policies to be followed in these situations. Where, then, does explaining the risks of medical radiation fit into the informed consent rubric? The Biological Effects of Ionizing Radiation (BEIR) VII report of the National Academy of Sciences states that 10 mSv of radiation exposure carries with it a 1 in 1000 chance of future malignancy in a 40-year-old adult [10]. This risk is considerably greater in children, approaching 1 in 100 in a 1-year-old girl [11].

At what level of risk estimate would it seem appropriate to actively provide information to patients? It may be appropriate to take guidance from risk estimates related to other medical procedures, which already employ informed consent in recognition of the morbidity and mortality associated with them. The rate of severe or fatal complications of endoscopic retrograde cholangiopancreatography (ERCP) was reported as low in experienced hands at a high-volume center, with 0.8% of severe complications and mortality of 0.08% [12]. Laparoscopic cholecystectomy, one of the most common surgical procedures performed in the USA, has a reported mortality rate of 0.3% and a rate of serious morbidity of 1.4% [13].

We believe that guidance could be obtained from works by the Veterans Health Administration (VHA) Directive 2008-002 on Disclosure of Adverse Events to Patients [14]. The VHA convened a multidisciplinary advisory board with representation from diverse stakeholder groups and experts, including physicians, nurses, and medical ethicists [14]. The board arrived at a risk estimate of 1 in 10,000; a risk greater than that required disclosure to patients, whereas a risk less than that did not require information. They did include the caveat that disclosure may still be warranted on the basis of ethical or other considerations. It should be noted that this determination was not created for medical radiation risks; however, at the same time this may be applicable for risks of all types in medical practice, including medical radiation.

There is controversy over the certitude of the risk estimates related to medical radiation [15], which no doubt contributes to the lack of general agreement that information should be provided to patients on radiation risks. The core of this controversy is the linear-no-threshold (LNT) risk model for estimation of radiation-related cancer cases. It should, however, be noted that this model is endorsed by all major radiation regulatory boards, including the International Commission on Radiological Protection (ICRP) [16], the National Academy of Sciences Committee on BEIR [17] and the United Nations Scientific Committee on the Effects of Atomic Radiation (UNSCEAR) [18], and also by the Food and Drug Administration (FDA) [19]. The BEIR VII executive summary states that "the risk of cancer proceeds in a linear fashion at lower doses without a threshold and that the smallest dose has the potential to cause a small increase in risk to humans" [10]. Low dose is defined by the BEIR VII committee as doses in the range of near zero up to about 100 mSv (0.1 Sv). Moreover, the great majority of published articles that directly examine medical radiation in a scientific fashion suggests a non-insignificant risk [20–23]. A recent article described a dose-dependent relationship between exposure to ionizing radiation from cardiac procedures, with a 3% increase in risk for cancer development over a mean follow-up period of 5 years for every additional 10 mSv experienced among a cohort of 82,861 patients [24].

In evaluating whether policies should be adopted, it is appropriate to consider what other developed nations are enacting.

In Europe, the Euratom law establishes that the need for an examination should be justified before a patient is referred to a radiologist or nuclear medicine physician, and a non-ionizing technique must be used whenever it will give grossly comparable information to an ionizing investigation [25]. It would appear prudent that the extent of information provided to patients regarding the risks of medical radiation, whether verbal or written consent, should vary with the dose/risk involved, and the patient [25]. Discussion of risks provides only half of the equation of forming a risk–benefit analysis. Description of benefits of the imaging test and risks of lack of disease detection, if the test is avoided, are also necessary.

There are many reasons for imaging specialists to be proactive in self-regulation, most of them self-evident and based upon our medical precept of *primum non nocere* (first do no harm). Experts in the discipline are better informed on the subject and hence better able to fashion regulations that are most prudent and appropriate. Open, respectful communication between health care provider and patient is an essential part of the physician–patient relationship. Patient-centered care is at the core of health care reform. Active information delivery serves to empower patients to be the stewards of their own health care. The present course of action, of doing relatively little, seems out of touch with modern health care. The lack of information delivery has been shown in studies that suggest that approximately 95% of patients are not informed of any radiation risk prior to their computed tomography (CT) scan [26, 27]. Actually, there has been limited improvement in the extent of information delivery on the risks of medical radiation since the prior study of Yale came out in 2006 [27], with a current study showing that only 24% of patients are informed of medical radiation risks [28].

If it is established that informed consent (either verbal or written) regarding the attendant risks of medical ionizing radiation should be performed, the next questions become:

1. Who should be consented?
2. At what radiation exposure is informed consent necessary?
3. What form of consent, verbal or written?
4. What source information should be used?
5. Who should do the consenting?

A reasonable concern for the radiologist and radiology practice is that if every medical radiation procedure requires informed consent, then the time commitment and resultant throughput impediments on health care workers and facilities will become prohibitively long. Mandatory written documentation of each patient's informed consent for every medical imaging procedure using ionizing radiation may result in both undue anxiety on the part of patients and occasional refusal by patients of procedures that may be necessary, and perhaps life-saving, when in fact the risk may be present but miniscule [29–31]. Our opinion is that provision of risk information in the informed consent process (whether verbal or written) should only be mandated for higher radiation dose procedures, and that perhaps 1 mSv is a prudent cutoff. Using 1 mSv as the threshold, procedures generally considered "high dose" such as CT, nuclear medicine tests, positron emission tomography (PET), PET–CT and fluoroscopic procedures (e.g. coronary angiography) would require this consent. Procedures generally considered "low dose," such as chest X-rays and X-rays of one bone region, would not require consent, as they are well below this threshold level and would not require information delivery of medical radiation risks.

The basis for selecting 1 mSv as the cutoff involves not only the simplicity of the number, and the fact that it separates low dose and high dose radiation procedures rather well, but also it is consistent with the VHA directive 2008-002 on Disclosure of Adverse Events to Patients (14). A risk of 1 in 10,000 corresponds fairly closely to a 1 mSv dose for a range of subjects; if the bar was set at 10 mSv instead, the risk would be at least 1 in 1000 for many subjects, and considerably greater in children. Additionally, 10 mSv is in the mid-range of CT exposures, as some CT procedures use less radiation (standard head CT) and some use more (chest and cardiac CT), and parsing out different CT procedures would be fraught with error.

Interestingly, our proposal for obtaining informed consent for exposures greater than 1 mSv was independently put forth by members of the International Atomic Energy Agency and select European imaging specialists with expertise in medical radiation safety [25].

The danger to the field of Radiology in not regulating itself and requiring informed consent for medical procedures using ionizing radiation is that we stand the very real chance of having regulations imposed upon us by government, as is already the case in Europe [25, 32]. The prospects of facing both poor public perception and imposed regulations is disturbing. The medical profession in general, and radiologists in particular, should not defer to government or the legal system to define parameters of informed consent (whether verbal or written) for radiation risk [33]. Although our opinion is that at least verbal informed consent detailing risks should be considered for all procedures of 1 mSv or greater, it is very likely this will be met with considerable resistance in the imaging community, and hence a good starting point may be requiring all imaging practices to actively provide information to patients undergoing "high dose" procedures by such means as distributing pamphlets on medical radiation risks to patients [34].

Additionally, an important part of the informed consent process (verbal and written) is the provision of information on alternate approaches, such as modalities that do not involve ionizing radiation, specifically ultrasound and magnetic resonance imaging (MRI); this discussion should reflect comparative effectiveness and comparative risk.

The obvious source material for information or medical radiation risk should be the National Academy of Sciences BEIR VII report [10]. Information derived from this is also available on the FDA website [15]. Our current recommendation is that presentation of information on risks and benefits may be conducted by radiologic technologists or radiologic physician assistants, with radiologists serving as backup. If actual consent is obtained, we think that initiating this approach with verbal consent may gain more acceptance among imaging specialists.

Lastly, a recently developed awareness campaign as a joint effort between the American College of Radiology (ACR) and the Radiological Society of North America entitled "Image Wisely" [35, 36], may be an ideal vehicle to promote the adoption of a strategy to provide information on medical radiation risk upon which patients then may give their consent to be imaged. The goal of the Image Wisely campaign is to ensure that patients undergo only radiation-based imaging examinations that are clinically indicated, and that they receive the lowest dose of radiation to generate diagnostic imaging studies (the as low as reasonably achievable [ALARA] principle) [35]. Although the first target audience will be imaging professionals, the campaign clearly identifies patients and the public as other important audiences. The Image Wisely campaign may be the ideal body to develop an information brochure that can be used by all imaging practices to distribute to patients undergoing "high dose" procedures.

We believe that the Radiology community should take the initiative to adopt guidelines and require that all imaging facilities use some form of active information process describing the risks of medical radiation [30].

Issues on imaging contrast media

Contrast agents have been in use for many years with the intent to improve medical imaging. Various clinical applications of imaging methods are directly dependent on administration of a contrast agent, as some examinations only exist because of that use (excluding intravenous urography, angiography, and others). Nonetheless, contrast agents, as any other pharmaceutical, carry a risk of an adverse event.

The radiologist's main roles regarding administration of contrast medium in a given imaging examination are: 1) to assure that the administration of contrast is appropriate for the patient and the indication; 2) to minimize the likelihood of a contrast reaction; and 3) to be fully prepared to treat a reaction should one occur [37].

Iodine contrast media

Today, about 80 to 90% of iodine-based contrast medium (ICM) is used for CT. Adverse reactions are infrequent and range from 5 to 12% for high osmolar ICM and from 1 to 3% for low osmolar ICM [16]. Moreover, most of these adverse reactions are mild, non-life-threatening events that usually require only observation, reassurance, and supportive measures, whereas the risk of a severe adverse drug reaction is about 0.2% for ionic ICM and 0.04% for non-ionic ICM; and the risk of a severe adverse drug reaction is 0.04% for ionic ICM and 0.004% for nonionic ICM [17]. Severe, sometimes life-threatening, adverse events occur unpredictably, most occurring immediately or within the first 20 minutes after contrast media injection. The majority of severe and very severe adverse reactions correspond to idiosyncratic reactions that are independent of the dose that is administered, and have been termed anaphylactoid, as they do not appear to be true anaphylaxis, but a similar phenomenon. Moreover, it is important to note that other complications following administration of ICM may occur, such as extravasation of a high volume of contrast with bolus injection technique, with related risks of skin sloughing and compartment syndrome.

Despite these risks, the ACR states that "Because of the documented low incidence of adverse events, intravenous injection of contrast media may be exempted from the need for informed consent, but this decision should be based on state law, institutional policy, and departmental policy" [37].

One of the most important complications related to ICM utilization is contrast induced-nephropathy (CIN). The definition of CIN includes three necessary components: 1) an absolute or relative increase in serum creatinine compared with the baseline values; 2) a temporal relationship between the rise in serum creatinine and exposure to a contrast agent; and 3) the exclusion of alternative explanations for renal failure [37, 38]. The exact pathophysiology of CIN is not completely understood [37]. Etiologic factors that have been suggested include: 1) renal hemodynamic changes (vasoconstriction), 2) direct tubular toxicity, and 3) high viscosity [37].

In the general population, the incidence of CIN is estimated to be 1 to 6% [39]. However, the risk may be as high as 50% in some patient subgroups. Patients with diabetes and preexisting renal impairment are at high risk, and CIN incidence increases in patients with multiple comorbidities. The volume and osmolality of contrast media used also play a role in the development of CIN. Patients who develop CIN are more likely to die in hospital and, for those who are discharged, 1-year mortality rates are high. Whether this is due to CM, comorbidity, or concurrent comorbid events is often unclear [39].

There is no specific therapy for CIN [42]. Thus, all efforts must be made to recognize patients at risk for CIN and to take appropriate preventive measures. There is evidence that patients at risk who received treatment with hydration before and after the administration of contrast have a lower rate of CIN. The standard hydration procedure involved intravenous infusion of isotonic saline (NaCl 0.9%) at a rate of 250 mL/hour for 4 hours before and 4 hours after exposure to contrast material [36]. Other treatments have been proposed, but to the present time no reproducible positive scientific confirmation has been shown [41, 42].

The most important risk factors for CIN are impaired renal function and diabetes mellitus [40]. Other risk factors include peripheral arterial disease, heart failure, age of more than 70 years, anemia, renal disease, renal surgery, proteinuria, hypertension, gout, administration of a large volume of contrast media, and use of diuretics, nonsteroidal anti-inflammatory drugs, or other nephrotoxic drugs [37, 40]. It is important to note that repeated administration within a 1-week period has increased risk. It is clear that older, high-osmolality ionic contrast media, such as diatrizoate and iothalamate, with osmolality values <1500 mOsm/kg, are more nephrotoxic than newer, low-osmolality contrast media (osmolality >900 mOsm/kg) [43], and as a result high-osmolar agent use has been abandoned in developed nations.

In practice, after ensuring that CT is necessary and contrast media should be used, the following should be established: 1) identification of

Table 5.1 Stages of renal diseases[†]

Stage	Description	GFR[*] (mL/min/1.73 m²)
1	Kidney damage with normal or increased GFR	≥90
2	Kidney damage with mildly decreased GFR	60–80
3	Moderately decreased GFR	30–59
4	Severely decreased GFR	15–29
5	Kidney failure	<15 (or dialysis)

Chronic kidney disease is defined as either kidney damage, or GFR lower than 60 mL/min/1.73 m² for more than 3 months.
[†]Glomerular filtration rate.
[*]The source is the National Kidney Foundation [46].

patients at risk; 2) stratification of these patients regarding renal function (to known estimated glomerular function rate [eGFR] less than 60 mL/min/1.73 m²) (Table 5.1); 3) promotion of treatment with hydration; 4) use of low or iso-osmolar contrast media; 5) use of the lowest dose of contrast medium consistent that will result in a diagnostic result; and 6) following of renal function of patients at risk (determine eGFR or serum creatinine) within 24 hours of contrast medium administration.

Gadolinium-based contrast media

Unlike with iodine contrast media, the risk of nephrotoxicity is very low when gadolinium-based contrast media (GBCM) are used in clinically approved doses. The major risk with GBCM is the development of nephrogenic systemic fibrosis (NSF).

NSF was first recognized in 1997, first described in the literature in 2000 [47], and first reported as a scleroderma-like fibrotic skin disorder seen exclusively in patients with renal insufficiency [47–52]. NSF may have systemic involvement that includes the heart, pericardium, pleura, diaphragm, kidneys, and testes [53–55]. It is characterized by increased deposits of collagen in tissues and most frequently involves the skin [56, 57]. The cutaneous findings of NSF include extensive thickening and hardening of the skin with hyperpigmentation; plaques, papules, and nodules; and a *peau d'orange* appearance [47–49]. Flexion contractures may occur around the joints and limit mobility [58, 59]. The severity of NSF varies; some patients may have mild disease, whereas others may have disease that progresses to severe patient debility, which may be fatal

[58, 60, 61]. Death usually is due to complications related to limited mobility and respiratory failure [60, 61].

Although the exact pathophysiology of NSF remains uncertain [50–52, 62–64], it does appear that leak of dissociated gadolinium into tissues induces a fibrogenic response that results in collagen deposition. Since mid-2006, reports have shown that the administration of gadolinium chelate contrast agents is associated with the development of NSF in patients with renal insufficiency [64–67]. In addition, free gadolinium has been detected in tissues affected by NSF [68, 69]. Thus, free gadolinium unbound from the chelating ligand has been suggested as an etiologic factor in the development of NSF [62, 70]. However, not all gadolinium chelate contrast agents have been reported to be associated with NSF, which relates to the stability of the chelate ligation among various GBCM available (Table 5.2) [64, 70, 71]. NSF has been associated predominantly with the use of gadodiamide, but it has also been reported in association with the administration of gadoversetamide and to a lesser likelihood gadopentetate dimeglumine [58, 64, 71].

Data from drug regulatory authorities and various registries (such as the Yale NSF Register) provide information on the number of patients who have been diagnosed with NSF [64]. Approximately 1600 cases have been reported to the FDA. Sixty hospitals in the USA account for 93% of these cases, and two hospitals in Denmark account for 4% of the cases [64]. Determining the true prevalence of NSF is, however, difficult [64]. It is likely that detection of the disease relates to the diligence of looking for it.

The GBCM-related risk factors are type of contrast and dose of contrast, whereas the patient-related risk factors are impaired renal function. Therefore, it is important to minimize the risk by identifying patients with high and intermediate risk, and when administration of contrast is necessary, use of the most stable contrast agents and lowest contrast dose are recommended.

Detailed recommendations and guidelines to minimize the risk of NSF can be found in selected references [37, 51, 64]. It should be recognized that the incidence of CIN with ICM is much higher than NSF with GBCM (Table 5.3) [40, 45, 63, 72]. It is not as well recognized that morbidity and mortality may not be so different between these entities, especially if CIN has resulted in the conversion of a patient from stage 3 renal failure to dialysis requiring stage 5 [73–76]. Our opinion is that whereas written informed consent is necessary for ICM administration in patients with stage 3 and greater renal failure, it is not the necessary for GBCM,

Table 5.2 The various commercially available gadolinium-based contrast agents and their characteristics

Name	Brand name	Chelate/ionicity	Viscosity mPa·s°	Osmolality mOsm/kg	Organ specific	Extracellular	Hepato-biliary	T½[a]	Relaxivity in plasma 1.5T – r_1 mM^{-1}s^{-1}[c]	Relaxivity in plasma 3.0 T – r_1 mM^{-1}s^{-1}[c]	Albumin binding	Stability	NSF risk[b]
Gadodiamide	Omniscan	Linear/non-ionic	1.4	780	No	Yes	No	1½h	4.3	4.0	No	Low	High
Gadoversetamide	Optimark	Linear/non-ioni	2.0	1,110	No	Yes	No	1½h	4.7	4.5	No	Low	High
Gadopentate dimeglumine	Magnevist	Linear/ionic	2.9	1,960	No	Yes	No	1½h	3.9–4.1	3.7–3.9	No	Intermediate	High
Gadopenate dimeglumine	Multihance	Linear/ionic	5.3	1,970	Yes (liver)	Mainly	Yes (1%–4%)	1½h	6.3–7.9	5.5–5.9	Yes (4%)	Intermediate	Intermediate
Gadoxetate disodium	Primovist, Eovist	Linear/ionic	1.2	688	Yes (liver)	No	Yes (42%–51%)	1½h	6.9	6.2	Yes (10%)	Intermediate	Intermediate
Gadofosveset trisodium	Vasovist, Ablavar	Linear/ionic	2.1	825	Yes (blood)	No	Yes (5%)	18h	19	9.9	Yes (90%)	Intermediate	Intermediate
Gadobutrol	Gadovist, Gadavist	Macrocyclic/non-ionic	5.0	1,603	No	Yes	No	1½h	4.7–5.2	4.5–5.0	No	High	Low
Gadoteridol	Prohance	Macrocyclic/non-ionic	1.3	630	No	Yes	No	1½h	4.1	3.7	No	High	Low
Gadoterate meglumine	Dotarem, Magnescope	Macrocyclic/non-ionic	2.0	1,350	No	Yes	No	1½h	3.6	3.5	No	High	Low

Taken from [71].

[a]In patients with normal renal function.

[b]According to the EMA classification.

[c]Determined at 37°C.

Table 5.3 Probabilistic risk estimates regarding CIN, NSF and exposure to radiation

CIN in renally impaired patients	1 in 5
NSF from Omniscan® in renally impaired patients	1 in 25
CIN in patients with normal renal function	1 in 50
Cancer from 10 mSv of radiation (one body CT)	1 in 1000
NSF from Omniscan®	1 in 2500
NSF from Magnevist®	1 in 40,000
Death from anaphylactoid reaction to non-ionic iodine contrast	1 in 130,000
Death from anaphylactoid reaction to gadolinium	1 in 280,000
NSF from MultiHance®	<1 in 4,000,000

provided stable agents are used for stage 3 and greater. Macrocyclic agents and agents with high biliary elimination (e.g.: MultiHance®, Eovist/Primovist®) are agents we recommend, and our preference is for low dose MultiHance® [77].

Ideal solution

The ideal solution would be to have comprehensive data on all diagnostic imaging procedures detailing risks, benefits, and costs, and relating these to their role for the investigation of major clinical entities. Many of the clinical scenarios do not permit controlled randomized prospective research studies; therefore, this limits our ability to provide absolute certainty regarding which is the best approach in all cases. An approach that we prefer to achieve accurate comparisons in imaging studies is cross-over design studies, in which all subjects receive both imaging approaches in a randomized cross-over fashion (i.e. first getting one and then getting the other). This has achieved success in MR contrast agent evaluation [78–80]. A complicating factor is that the current speed of development/use of new drugs, new diagnostic procedures (even within the same imaging modality considering new protocols, sequences, and techniques), and new therapeutic options, exceed our capacity of scientific investigation, at least of our ability to keep pace with developments. Thus, there exists, and likely will always exist, a time lag between innovation and evaluation with comparative-effectiveness approaches of scientifically assessed value. A major limitation is also funding, as funding is generally not readily available to do clinical comparisons in a randomized fashion between imaging strategies. Funding is often challenging in clinical imaging research, and imaging studies are in general very costly, so funds would need to be set aside, by federal funding agencies, to support comparative-effectiveness research between imaging modalities by credible researchers. This type of research has generally been considered too mundane to achieve interest by the National Institutes of Health.

Solving the funding issues and thereby gaining access to comparative data (including data that compare with no imaging at all) that is meaningful, radiologists can then provide truly well-informed and scientific risk–benefit analyses to patients.

Shared decision making

The key features of shared decision making are: 1) the involvement of at least two participants, the physician and the patient; 2) information shared between both parties; 3) steps by both parties to build a consensus about the preferred treatment; and 4) an agreement reached on the treatment to implement [81]. Although it is recognized that shared decision making may not work for all types of patients or clinical situations, it has gained a high level of policy support and ultimately does produce beneficial results as shown by evidence-based data [82–84].

The concept of shared decision making intertwines all aspects of medical management (i.e. diagnosis, treatment, and follow-up options). A noteworthy example of this is shared decision making concerning the option of active surveillance for men diagnosed with low-risk prostate cancer [85]. The value of this is that low-risk prostate cancer shows a low growth potential and therefore is likely to remain clinically asymptomatic during the lifetime of an individual [85], hence differing subjects may have a different risk tolerance for this uncertain but unlikely outcome. A recently published study described 731 men with localized prostate cancer, randomly assigned to either surgery or observation [86]. During the median follow-up of 10.0 years, 171 of 364 men (47.0%) assigned to radical prostatectomy died, compared with 183 of 367 (49.9%) assigned to observation (hazard ratio, 0.88; 95% confidence interval [CI], 0.71 to 1.08; $P = 0.22$; absolute risk reduction, 2.9 percentage points). Among men assigned to radical prostatectomy, 21 (5.8%) died from prostate cancer or treatment, compared with 31 men (8.4%) assigned to observation (hazard ratio, 0.63; 95% CI, 0.36 to 1.09; $P = 0.09$; absolute risk reduction, 2.6 percentage points). The effect of treatment on all-cause and prostate-cancer mortality did not differ according to age, race, coexisting conditions, self-reported performance status, or histologic features of the tumor. Radical prostatectomy was associated with reduced all-cause mortality among men with a prostate-specific antigen (PSA) value greater than 10 ng/mL (P = 0.04 for interaction) and possibly among those with intermediate-risk or high-risk tumors (P = 0.07 for interaction). Adverse events within 30 days after surgery occurred in 21.4% of men, including one death [86]. They concluded that among men with localized prostate cancer detected during the early era of PSA testing, radical prostatectomy did not significantly reduce all-cause or prostate-cancer mortality, compared with observation, through at least 12 years of follow-up [86]. The patient then has to weigh their acceptability of a slightly greater short-term risk of death from treatment, against a slightly better long-term outlook. In another recent report, it was concluded that in order to facilitate a more patient-oriented decision-making process regarding treatment in those with clinically localized prostate cancer, clinicians need to tailor their interventions according to patient age and cancer aggressiveness, help reduce patient concerns and misconceptions regarding the physical impact of treatments, allow sufficient time for patients to consider treatment options, and assist patients in balancing advice and information received from different sources [87]. Current data show that there are more men choosing to live with cancer in place, rather than the standard "get it out" surgical approach, with added benefit of quality of life.

Anecdotal descriptions and lack of controlled comparisons should be avoided in all of health care, but also in imaging as well. However, anecdotal experience is widely touted in the lay press. A case in point: one subject who had a radical prostatectomy at age 50 for prostate cancer disputed the current recommendation by the government US Preventive Services Task Force (USPSTF) that routine PSA screening is not indicated in men over 50, claiming that he would not be alive if it was not for this screening [88]. Of course the obvious flaw, overlooked by the media, is that there is no controlled comparison of how he would have done without the prostatectomy, and the answer is probably better. The simple answer is beware of anecdotes in all their forms; they are often driven by the bias of validating individual choices, and have essentially no scientific merit. To contribute to achieving more balanced large population data, and information based upon this, detailed information and research results data are available through many legitimate websites, such as the Prostate Cancer Foundation (http://www.pcf.org/). This represents one example of an area of active and directed research with evidence being sought to build solid scientific evidence on a specific disease process, with the purpose of shedding light on optimal treatment approaches. Of course this goal is far from complete for prostate cancer, as there are so many questions unanswered on comparative effectiveness, including on the role of various imaging modalities. However, the point is that it is essential to establish databases that provide large population-based outcome results for various strategies of treatment. Our goal would be to have this outcome data available for imaging studies, where the outcome measurements evaluated include the composite of harm related to the procedure, and the quality and length of life in general.

There are many shared-decision-making topics that concern radiological practice, although most of these decisions are made one step earlier in the health care process, in the discussion between the primary physician and the patient. Indeed, much of the radiologists' role in this shared-decision-making equation is in their role in educating physicians, such as in the setting of clinical rounds and multidisciplinary conferences, at which the optimal diagnostic imaging exams and procedures are discussed for each given case. More comprehensive discussion of this subject of referring physician education is presented in Chapter 6. Graduate and postgraduate medical curricula must also include information on radiology appropriateness and diagnostic performance issues—that is, the best indications for each imaging method, the contraindications, the costs, and the risks (e.g. radiation, contrast agents, pre-exam preparations).

Workable solution

The workable solution is to combine information available from major research-driven publications, marketing information from companies, and experience from experts. All of these sources, however, must be rigorously evaluated for impartiality, which may be an unrealizable goal; therefore, prudent judgment and skepticism are advised. Over recent years major companies in Radiology have been held accountable for their false marketing claims, and various federal agencies have pursued the requirement of companies to show integrity in their marketing material. This affects the integrity of not only those punished, but also of other competitor companies, as they will want to avoid punitive measures themselves.

In advancing the reliability of information, physicians are better positioned to discuss risk–benefit analyses with patients. This risk–benefit discussion should be mandated for circumstances in which the risk is considered "likely to be real." For medical radiation, we consider this to be imaging tests where the radiation exposure is estimated to be greater than 1 mSv.

Almost as much as with medical radiation, accurate information about contrast agent risks is also sparse. Using the number established by the VA health directive described above, in circumstances where risk for serious injury exceeds an expected 1 in 10,000 likelihood, then that risk ought to be discussed with the patient. Contrast agent risks have been estimated and presented in Table 5.3. As the table reveals, the risk for contrast-induced nephropathy due to iodine contrast used in CT in patients in chronic renal failure stage 3 is much greater, at 5%, than for NSF with stable agents (MultiHance®, Prohance®, Gadavist®) for stage 3 where the risk approaches 0%, but also for stage 4 (also close to 0%), and possibly even for stage 5. Our recommendation, though, is to do careful risk–benefit evaluation for stage 5.

As a starting point, it may be easiest to provide brochures to patients when they check in, to read as they are waiting, and the technologists can answer questions, or direct the patient to radiologists if this is beyond the scope of the technologist. Ultimately, it may be necessary to acquire written consent approval; however, we would not advocate that for procedures where the radiation exposure is <1 mSv or for contrast agents where for the particular patient the risk of a serious adverse outcome is <1 in 10,000.

References

1. Semelka RC, Armao DM, Elias J, Jr, et al. The information imperative: Is it time for an informed consent process explaining the risks of medical radiation? Radiology 2012; 262:15–8.
2. Edwards A, Elwyn G. Shared decision-making in healthcare: achieving evidence-based patient choice. In: Edwards A, Elwyn G, eds. Shared decision-making in health care. Achieving evidence-based patient choice. 2nd ed. New York: Oxford University Press Inc., 2009; pp. 3–10.
3. Cobbs v. Grant, 8 Cal. 3d 229, 502 P.2d 1, 104 Cal. Rptr. 505 (1972).
4. Canterbury v. Spence, 150 U.S. App. D.C. 263, 464 F.2d 772 (1972).
5. Reuter SR. An overview of informed consent for radiologists. AJR Am J Roentgenol 1987; 148:219–227.
6. Mavroforou A, Giannoukas A, Mavrophoros D, et al. Physicians' liability in interventional radiology and endovascular therapy. Eur J Radiol 2003; 46:240–243.
7. O'Dwyer HM, Lyon SM, Fotheringham T, et al. Informed consent for interventional radiology procedures: A survey detailing current European practice. Cardiovasc Intervent Radiol 2003; 26:428–433.
8. Phatouros CC, Blake MP. How much now to tell? Patients' attitudes to an information sheet prior to angiography and angioplasty. Australas Radiol 1995; 39:135–139.

9. Brenner DJ, Hricak H. Radiation exposure from medical imaging: Time to regulate? JAMA 2010; 304:208–209.

10. BEIR-VII. Executive Summary. In: Board on Radiation Effects Research - Division on Earth and Life Studies editor. Health Risks from Exposure to Low Levels of Ionizing Radiation: BEIR VII – Phase 2. Washington, D.C.: The National Academy Press, 2005.

11. Brenner D, Elliston C, Hall E, et al. Estimated risks of radiation-induced fatal cancer from pediatric CT. AJR Am J Roentgenol 2001; 176:289–296.

12. Salminen P, Laine S, Gullichsen R. Severe and fatal complications after ERCP: Analysis of 2555 procedures in a single experienced center. Surg Endosc 2008; 22:1965–1970.

13. Ingraham AM, Cohen ME, Ko CY, et al. A current profile and assessment of North American cholecystectomy: Results from the american college of surgeons national surgical quality improvement program. J Am Coll Surg 2011; 211:176–186.

14. Veterans Health Administration. Disclosure of adverse events to patients. VHA directive 2008-002. Washington, DC: Department of Veterans Affairs, January 18, 2008. Available online at: http://www1.va.gov/vhapublications/viewpublication.asp?pub_id=1637. [accessed April 23, 2013].

15. Brant-Zawadzki M. Diagnostic radiology: Major weapon in patient care or weapon of mass destruction? J Am Coll Radiol 2005; 2:301–303.

16. 1990 Recommendations of the International Commission on Radiological Protection. Ann ICRP 1991; 21:1–201.

17. Committee on the Biological Effects of Ionizing Radiation (BEIR V) NRC: Health Effects of Exposure to Low Levels of Ionizing Radiation: BEIR V. Washington, DC: National Academy Press, 1990.

18. UNSCEAR 2000 Report to the General Assembly. In: United Nations Scientific Committee on the Effects of Atomic Radiation 2000.

19. FDA. What are the Radiation Risks from CT? U.S. Food and Drug Administration 2005. Available online at: http://www.fda.gov/ForConsumers/ConsumerUpdates/ucm115329.htm. [accessed March 5, 2013].

20. Einstein AJ, Weiner SD, Bernheim A, et al. Multiple testing, cumulative radiation dose, and clinical indications in patients undergoing myocardial perfusion imaging. JAMA 2010; 304:2137–2144.

21. Rajaraman P, Simpson J, Neta G, et al. Early life exposure to diagnostic radiation and ultrasound scans and risk of childhood cancer: Case-control study. BMJ 2011; 342:d472.

22. Berrington de Gonzalez A, Darby S. Risk of cancer from diagnostic X-rays: Estimates for the UK and 14 other countries. Lancet 2004; 363:345–351.

23. Smith-Bindman R, Lipson J, Marcus R, et al. Radiation dose associated with common computed tomography examinations and the associated lifetime attributable risk of cancer. Arch Intern Med 2009; 169:2078–2086.

24. Eisenberg MJ, Afilalo J, Lawler PR, et al. Cancer risk related to low-dose ionizing radiation from cardiac imaging in patients after acute myocardial infarction. CMAJ 2011; 183:430–436.

25. Malone J, Guliera R, Craven C, et al. Justification of diagnostic medical exposures: some practical issues. Report of an International Atomic Energy Agency Consultation. Br J Radiol 2012; 85: 523–538.

26. Andrieu N, Easton DF, Chang-Claude J, et al. Effect of chest X-rays on the risk of breast cancer among BRCA1/2 mutation carriers in the international BRCA1/2 carrier cohort study: A report from the EMBRACE, GENEPSO, GEO-HEBON, and IBCCS Collaborators' Group. J Clin Oncol 2006; 24:3361–3366.

27. Lee CI, Flaster HV, Haims AH, et al. Diagnostic CT scans: institutional informed consent guidelines and practices at academic medical centers. Am J Roentgenol 2006; 187:282–287.

28. Caverly TJ, Prochazka AV, Cook-Shimanek M, et al. Weighing the Potential Harms of Computed Tomography: Patient Survey. JAMA Intern Med 2013:1–2.

29. Dudzinski DM, Hebert PC, Foglia MB, et al. The disclosure dilemma—large-scale adverse events. N Engl J Med 2010; 363:978–986.

30. Hendee WR, Becker GJ, Borgstede JP, et al. Addressing overutilization in medical imaging. Radiology 2010; 257:240–245.

31. Vartanians VM, Sistrom CL, Weilburg JB, Rosenthal DI, Thrall JH. Increasing the appropriateness of outpatient imaging: effects of a barrier to ordering low-yield examinations. Radiology 2010; 255:842–849.

32. Picano E. Informed consent and communication of risk from radiological and nuclear medicine examinations: how to escape from a communication inferno. BMJ 2004; 329:849–851.

33. Baerlocher MO, Detsky AS. Discussing radiation risks associated with CT scans with patients. JAMA 2010; 304:2170–2171.

34. Coakley FV, Gould R, Yeh BM, et al. CT radiation dose: What can you do right now in your practice? AJR Am J Roentgenol 2011; 196:619–625.

35. Brink JA, Amis ES, Jr. Image Wisely: A campaign to increase awareness about adult radiation protection. Radiology 2010; 257:601–602.

36. Martino A. Patient safety: Road map to Imaging Wisely. ACR Bulletin 2010; 65:7.

37. ACR Committee on Drugs and Contrast Media. ACR Manual on Contrast Media, 2012.

38. Bush WH, Swanson DP. Acute reactions to intravascular contrast media: types, risk factors, recognition, and specific treatment. AJR Am J Roentgenol 1991; 157:1153–1161.

39. Katayama H, Yamaguchi K, Kozuka T, Takashima T, Seez P, Matsuura K. Adverse reactions to ionic and nonionic contrast media. A report from the Japanese Committee on the Safety of Contrast Media. Radiology 1990; 175:621–628.

40. Mehran R, Nikolsky E. Contrast-induced nephropathy: Definition, epidemiology, and patients at risk. Kidney Int Suppl 2006:S11–15.

41. Parfrey P. The clinical epidemiology of contrast-induced nephropathy. Cardiovasc Intervent Radiol 2005; 28 Suppl 2:S3–11.

42. Balemans CE, Reichert LJ, van Schelven BI, et al. Epidemiology of contrast material-induced nephropathy in the era of hydration. Radiology 2012; 263:706–713.

43. Albabtain MA, Almasood A, Alshurafah H, et al. Efficacy of ascorbic acid, N-Acetylcysteine, or combination of both on top of saline hydration versus saline hydration alone on prevention of contrast-induced nephropathy: A prospective randomized study. J Interv Cardiol 2012; 26:90–96.

44. Marenzi G, Cabiati A, Milazzo V, Rubino M. Contrast-induced nephropathy. Intern Emerg Med 2012; 7 Suppl 3:181–183.

45. Solomon R, Dumouchel W. Contrast media and nephropathy: Findings from systematic analysis and Food and Drug Administration reports of adverse effects. Invest Radiol 2006; 41:651–660.
46. Levey AS, Coresh J, Balk E, et al. National Kidney Foundation practice guidelines for chronic kidney disease: evaluation, classification, and stratification. Ann Intern Med 2003; 139:137–147.
47. Cowper SE, Robin HS, Steinberg SM, Su LD, Gupta S, LeBoit PE. Scleromyxoedema-like cutaneous diseases in renal-dialysis patients. Lancet 2000; 356:1000–1001.
48. Cowper SE. Nephrogenic fibrosing dermopathy: The first 6 years. Curr Opin Rheumatol 2003; 15:785–790.
49. Cowper SE, Su LD, Bhawan J, et al. Nephrogenic fibrosing dermopathy. Am J Dermatopathol 2001; 23:383–393.
50. Altun E, Martin DR, Wertman R, Lugo-Somolinos A, Fuller ER, 3rd, Semelka RC. Nephrogenic systemic fibrosis: change in incidence following a switch in gadolinium agents and adoption of a gadolinium policy-report from two U.S. universities. Radiology 2009; 253:689–696.
51. Altun E, Semelka RC, Cakit C. Nephrogenic systemic fibrosis and management of high-risk patients. Acad Radiol 2009; 16:897–905
52. Wertman R, Altun E, Martin DR, et al. Risk of nephrogenic systemic fibrosis: Evaluation of gadolinium chelate contrast agents at four American universities. Radiology 2008; 248:799–806.
53. Daram SR, Cortese CM, Bastani B. Nephrogenic fibrosing dermopathy/nephrogenic systemic fibrosis: Report of a new case with literature review. Am J Kidney Dis 2005; 46:754–759.
54. Gibson SE, Farver CF, Prayson RA. Multiorgan involvement in nephrogenic fibrosing dermopathy: An autopsy case and review of the literature. Arch Pathol Lab Med 2006; 130:209–212.
55. Kucher C, Steere J, Elenitsas R, et al. Nephrogenic fibrosing dermopathy/nephrogenic systemic fibrosis with diaphragmatic involvement in a patient with respiratory failure. J Am Acad Dermatol 2006; 54:S31–34.
56. Galan A, Cowper SE, Bucala R. Nephrogenic systemic fibrosis (nephrogenic fibrosing dermopathy). Curr Opin Rheumatol 2006; 18:614–617.
57. Mendoza FA, Artlett CM, Sandorfi N, et al. Description of 12 cases of nephrogenic fibrosing dermopathy and review of the literature. Semin Arthritis Rheum 2006; 35:238–249.
58. Kuo PH, Kanal E, Abu-Alfa AK, et al. Gadolinium-based MR contrast agents and nephrogenic systemic fibrosis. Radiology 2007; 242:647–649.
59. Romanelli P, Bouzari N. New clinical syndromes in dermatology. Semin Cutan Med Surg 2006; 25:79–86.
60. Evenepoel P, Zeegers M, Segaert S, et al. Nephrogenic fibrosing dermopathy: A novel, disabling disorder in patients with renal failure. Nephrol Dial Transplant 2004; 19:469–473.
61. Sadowski EA, Bennett LK, Chan MR, et al. Nephrogenic systemic fibrosis: Risk factors and incidence estimation. Radiology 2007; 243:148–157.
62. Grobner T. Gadolinium-a specific trigger for the development of nephrogenic fibrosing dermopathy and nephrogenic systemic fibrosis? Nephrol Dial Transplant 2006; 21:1104–1108.

63. Lauenstein TC, Salman K, Morreira R, et al. Nephrogenic systemic fibrosis: Center case review. J Magn Reson Imaging 2007; 26:1198–1203.

64. Thomsen HS, Morcos SK, Almen T, et al. Nephrogenic systemic fibrosis and gadolinium-based contrast media: Updated ESUR Contrast Medium Safety Committee guidelines. Eur Radiol 2013; 23:307–318.

65. FDA. Magnevist - Label and Approval History. U.S. Department of Health and Human Services Food and Drug Administration 2006. Available online at: http://www.accessdata.fda.gov/scripts/cder/drugsatfda/index.cfm?fuseaction=Search. Label_ApprovalHistory. [accessed March 5, 2013].

66. FDA. Public Health Advisory–Gadolinium-containing contrast agents for magnetic resonance imaging (MRI). U.S. Food and Drug Administration 2006. Available online at: http://www.fda.gov/Drugs/DrugSafety/PostmarketDrugSafetyInformation forPatientsandProviders/DrugSafetyInformationforHeathcareProfessionals/ PublicHealthAdvisories/ucm053112.htm [accessed March 5, 2013].

67. Marckmann P, Skov L, Rossen K, et al. Nephrogenic systemic fibrosis: Suspected causative role of gadodiamide used for contrast-enhanced magnetic resonance imaging. J Am Soc Nephrol 2006; 17:2359–2362.

68. High WA, Ayers RA, Chandler J, et al. Gadolinium is detectable within the tissue of patients with nephrogenic systemic fibrosis. J Am Acad Dermatol 2007; 56:21–26.

69. White GW, Gibby WA, Tweedle MF. Comparison of Gd(DTPA-BMA) (Omniscan) versus Gd(HP-DO3A) (ProHance) relative to gadolinium retention in human bone tissue by inductively coupled plasma mass spectroscopy. Invest Radiol 2006; 41:272–278.

70. Lin SP, Brown JJ. MR contrast agents: Physical and pharmacologic basics. J Magn Reson Imaging 2007; 25:884–899.

71. Thomsen HS, Marckmann P. Extracellular Gd-CA: Differences in prevalence of NSF. Eur J Radiol 2008; 66:180–183.

72. Thomsen HS, Marckmann P, Logager VB. Enhanced computed tomography or magnetic resonance imaging: A choice between contrast medium-induced nephropathy and nephrogenic systemic fibrosis? Acta Radiol 2007; 48:593–596.

73. Levy EM, Viscoli CM, Horwitz RI. The effect of acute renal failure on mortality. A cohort analysis. JAMA 1996; 275:1489–1494.

74. McCullough PA, Adam A, Becker CR, et al. Epidemiology and prognostic implications of contrast-induced nephropathy. Am J Cardiol 2006; 98:5K–13K.

75. McCullough PA, Stacul F, Becker CR, et al. Contrast-Induced Nephropathy (CIN) Consensus Working Panel: Executive summary. Rev Cardiovasc Med 2006; 7:177–197.

76. Stacul F, Adam A, Becker CR, et al. Strategies to reduce the risk of contrast-induced nephropathy. Am J Cardiol 2006; 98:59K–77K.

77. de Campos RO, Heredia V, Ramalho M, et al. Quarter-dose (0.025 mmol/kg) gadobenate dimeglumine for abdominal MRI in patients at risk for nephrogenic systemic fibrosis: Preliminary observations. AJR Am J Roentgenol 2011; 196:545–552.

78. Bueltmann E, Erb G, Kirchin MA, et al. Intra-individual crossover comparison of gadobenate dimeglumine and gadopentetate dimeglumine for contrast-enhanced

magnetic resonance angiography of the supraaortic vessels at 3 Tesla. Invest Radiol 2008; 43:695–702.

79. Maravilla KR, Maldjian JA, Schmalfuss IM, et al. Contrast enhancement of central nervous system lesions: multicenter intraindividual crossover comparative study of two MR contrast agents. Radiology 2006; 240:389–400.

80. Colosimo C, Knopp MV, Barreau X, et al. A comparison of Gd-BOPTA and Gd-DOTA for contrast-enhanced MRI of intracranial tumours. Neuroradiology 2004; 46:655–665.

81. Charles C, Gafni A, Whelan T. Shared decision-making in the medical encounter: What does it mean? (or it takes at least two to tango). Soc Sci Med 1997; 44:681–692.

82. Crawford MJ, Rutter D, Manley C, et al. Systematic review of involving patients in the planning and development of health care. BMJ 2002; 325:1263.

83. O'Connor AM, Bennett CL, Stacey D, et al. Decision aids for people facing health treatment or screening decisions. Cochrane Database Syst Rev 2009:CD001431.

84. Legare F, Turcotte S, Stacey D, et al. Patients' perceptions of sharing in decisions: A systematic review of interventions to enhance shared decision making in routine clinical practice. Patient 2012; 5:1–19.

85. Bangma CH, Bul M, van der Kwast TH, et al. Active surveillance for low-risk prostate cancer. Crit Rev Oncol Hematol 2013; 85:295–302.

86. Wilt TJ, Brawer MK, Jones KM, et al. Radical prostatectomy versus observation for localized prostate cancer. N Engl J Med 2012; 367:203–213.

87. Prostate Cancer Foundation. Available online at: http://www.pcf.org. [accessed March 5, 2013].

88. Walker EP. PSA screening for prostate cancer debated in Congress. Available online at: http://www.kevinmd.com/blog/2010/03/defending-psa-screening-prostate-cancer-congress.html [accessed February 27, 2013].

CHAPTER 6

Are we doing the right study?

Diane Armao,[1] Jorge Elias Jr,[2] and Richard C. Semelka[3]

[1] University of North Carolina at Chapel Hill, School of Medicine, Department of Radiology and Pathology and Laboratory Medicine, Chapel Hill, NC, USA
[2] The School of Medicine of Ribeirao Preto, University of Sao Paulo, Brazil
[3] University of North Carolina at Chapel Hill, School of Medicine, Department of Radiology, Chapel Hill, NC, USA

This chapter complements and expands issues discussed in Chapter 2. The rapid rise of medical imaging reflects ongoing advances in technology and expanded applications in high-tech modalities. This growth rate is abetted by reflexive acceptance of imaging as standard of care, without an evidence base to create formal practice guidelines. In this chapter we describe the current status of tools such as computer-based clinical decision support, which should serve the critical goal of ensuring that appropriate imaging studies are being performed, while inappropriate studies are avoided.

Introduction

That there is immense waste in US health care spending is inarguable. Wasteful spending in the health care system has been calculated at up to $1.2 trillion of the $2.2 trillion spent nationally, more than half of all health care costs [1]. "Waste" may be defined as costs that could have been avoided without a negative impact on quality of care [1]. Crucial players in driving up the price of excess include culture, politics, profit and incentives, medicolegal liability, and lack of a coordinated focus. Solving the problem of excess spending involves creating system-wide incentives that encourage partnership, and networks that aim for shared value. When compared with other industrialized nations, the USA spends nearly twice as much per capita on health care, yet ranks at the bottom of key health system efficiency measures, including life expectancy, infant

Health Care Reform in Radiology, First Edition. Richard C. Semelka and Jorge Elias Jr.
© 2013 John Wiley & Sons, Inc. Published 2013 by John Wiley & Sons, Inc.

mortality, obesity, and avoidable deaths [2]. Abundant sources of inefficiencies obtain in US health care, ranging from administrative complexity, lack of price information and incentives for patients, as well as scientific uncertainty about effectiveness and costs, especially of newer tests and treatments [3, 4]. A recently released report by the Institute of Medicine (IOM) "Best care at lower cost: The path to continuously learning health care in America" [5] cautions health care providers that as advances in health care are embraced, one must also remember that a number of what were thought to be advances turned out not to be beneficial, but were, instead, even harmful tests and treatments [4].

Medical imaging's image: More and more is less and less

Over the past decade, dramatic increases in the use of diagnostic imaging have contributed to soaring medical costs and medical exposure to ionizing radiation [6]. Recent summary statements from the Medicare Payment Advisory Commission (MedPAC) to the Centers for Medicare and Medicaid Services (CMS) reported that the rise in volume of medical services per Medicare beneficiary outstripped the growth of all other services that physicians provide [7]. For example, between 2000 and 2005, spending for imaging more than doubled from $6.6 billion to $13.7 billion, an average growth rate twice the overall rate of growth in physician fee schedule services [8]. Costs for diagnostic imaging are among the fastest growing Medicare expenses, and imaging costs among Medicare beneficiaries with cancer increased from 1999 through 2006, outpacing the rate of increase in total costs among Medicare beneficiaries with cancer [9]. Notably, diagnostic imaging ordering intensity is not limited to Medicare and fee-for-service models of care. A recent, large, multisite study assessing trends in integrated health care delivery systems, or health maintenance organizations (HMOs), that are fiscally accountable for the outcomes and health status of the population served, describe similar patterns of increasing utilization [10]. For example, within six large HMOs using bundled payments for imaging services, overall computed tomography (CT) use tripled from about 50 tests per 1000 patients in 1996, to 150 per 1000 patients in 2012, while magnetic resonance imaging (MRI) scans quadrupled from 17 per 1000 patients to 65 per 1000 patients over the same period [10]. In the past decade, diagnostic imaging services and their costs have increased at twice the rate of other health care technologies, including laboratory procedures and pharmaceuticals [11]. Despite ever-rising expenditures for imaging services, estimated at $100 billion annually [10], data that documents a close connection between most diagnostic imaging procedures and patients' outcomes are lacking [12].

Some publications have suggested that up to 20–50% of high-tech imaging, such as multisection CT, MRI, and positron emission tomography (PET), fail to provide information that improves patients' welfare and hence may represent unnecessary imaging services [11]. By definition, *overutilization* may be defined as application of imaging procedures in clinical situations where imaging tests are unlikely to improve patient outcomes [11]. Inappropriate imaging augments health care costs without increasing the quality of health care. Recent research shows that approximately one-third of health care spending is duplicative or unhelpful, or makes patients worse [13]. Seminal research involving wide variation in Medicare spending in different regions of the USA revealed that Medicare enrollees in high-spending areas did not receive better quality care, improved access to care or better health outcomes and patient satisfaction [14]. In fact, the greater than twofold differences observed across US regions, $8414 per enrollee in the Miami region compared with $3341 in the Minneapolis region, are not due to differences in the average levels of illness or socioeconomic status [14]. Rather, as the researchers poignantly point out, cost variations are due to the overall quantity of medical services provided and the predominance of subspecialists in high-cost regions [14]. Unnecessary imaging studies seldom reveal the cause of the patients' complaint, yet may reveal incidental findings that require further imaging or interventional procedures to clarify [15].

The rapid rise of medical imaging reflects ongoing advances in technology and expanded applications in high-tech modalities. This growth rate is abetted by reflexive acceptance of imaging as standard of care, without an evidence base to create formal practice guidelines. In a *New England Journal of Medicine* (NEJM) perspective piece, and fine example of literary apostrophe, entitled "Waste, we know you are out there," the director of the Congressional Budget Office is cited as stating "a variety of credible evidence suggests that health care contains the largest inefficiencies in our economy. As much as $700 billion a year in health care services are delivered in the U.S. that do not improve health outcomes" [16]. Reports teem of inappropriate, low-yield, low-benefit procedures. Yet there exists a permissiveness within the current health care system and imaging community fueled by a complex array of causative factors, including: 1) the knowledge gap of the ordering provider and lack of support in the appropriate clinical application of diagnostic imaging [17, 18]; 2) technical advances that have led to expansion of clinical applications [10]; 3) patient- and physician-generated demand [10]; 4) intolerance of diagnostic uncertainty [18]; 5) defensive medicine, accounting for approximately 1 in 5 examinations [19]; 6) inaccessibility or ignorance of previously performed examinations, which is estimated at approximately 1 in 5 examinations [20]; 7) imaging as a surrogate for physical examination, a practice most marked in the emergency room setting [18]; 8) financially motivated self-referral and radiologists' imaging recommendations for repeat studies [18]; and 9) the paramount, pervasive all-too-human factor associated with the mindless repetition of established routine—"That's the way we do it here" [16]. Such evidence counters popular belief that technological advances and more spending will result in improved health care quality, meanwhile pressing home the ponderous reality of health care waste.

As a case in point, a very recent study published in the *Journal of the National Cancer Institute* and utilizing claims within the Surveillance, Epidemiology and End Results (SEER)-Medicare database between 1994 and 2009, indicates that the use of high cost advanced diagnostic imaging including CT, MRI, PET, and nuclear medicine is growing faster among patients with stage IV breast, colorectal, lung, and prostate cancer than it is among patients with earlier stages of disease [21]. In this study, Hu et al. report that for patients with stage IV cancer diagnosed between 2002 and 2006, the mean and median number of high-cost imaging procedures per patient were 9.6 and 7, respectively [21]. The investigators state "Because scans help clinicians determine whether a change in (or cessation of) treatment is indicated, the expanding use of advanced imaging in stage IV disease is likely a manifestation of the increasing number and types of treatment options available to these patients" [21]. Important note is made of the fact that for the four tumor types studied, survival in incident stage IV disease "has changed modestly, if at all, over the past one or two decades; although treatment may be changing (and imaging with it), the natural history of metastatic disease is not" [21]. This emphasizes one of our major concerns, that more and more health care expenditure is directed at the care of individuals in the terminal stages of their lives, who are the least likely to show appreciable or measurable benefit from it.

In the setting of advanced disease, guidelines attempting to define the role of advanced imaging are few. Currently, routine use of imaging is recommended by the National Comprehensive Cancer Network (NCCN) only in patients with colorectal cancer metastatic to the lung or liver [22]. In sharp contrast, national practice guidelines have been recently established for a circumscribed role in imaging in the post-treatment surveillance of patients with early stage breast, lung, colorectal, and prostate cancer in response to evolving evidence of its limited utility in these settings [21]. Routine advanced imaging is now recommended only in lung and select colon cancer patients. Correspondingly, in the study's cohort of patients with stage I and stage II disease, the frequency and intensity of imaging outside of the diagnostic period declined over time.

In the midst of a national thrust for cost-effectiveness and evidence-based outcomes research, the need for high-tech imaging guidelines during terminal illness care is imperative. Editorialists reviewing the results of research by Hu et al. state that " In the United Kingdom, the National Institute for Clinical Excellence, the organization that evaluates both medical and economic evidence for the National Health Service, has issued 'do not do' recommendations for some high-cost imaging in patients with advanced cancer" [23]. Further commentary addresses the need for clinical decision support algorithms embedded within the electronic medical record within the context of patient-centered care during terminal stages of disease. Finally, as the research team of Hu et al. presciently point out, "Imaging, although it often leads to (appropriate) palliative measures, may also distract patients from focusing on achievable end-of-life goals, require them to spend more of their limited time in medical care settings, and/or provoke anxiety" [21].

The fragmentation of US medical care is oftentimes highlighted in care that terminally ill patients receive, which frequently exerts a deep and enduring personal toll on both patients and their loved ones. Some key concepts were openly addressed in a narrative published in *Newsweek* by Anne Bennett regarding her husband's high cost of end-of-life care [24]. Ms. Bennett states "The system masks all kinds of agendas—from the desire to live to the desire to turn a profit—that makes the choices for us infinitely more complex. Confusion, lack of coordination and lack of oversight yield expensive overtreatment—but not necessarily better care." The author recalls her husband having "many CT scans—I might have guessed two dozen over the years. The actual number was 76, more than 10 a year for 7 years." In the same article, palliative care specialist physician Ira Byock argues that overtreatment is an unfortunate side effect of medical advances. "We have enormous scientific prowess and remarkable diagnostics and treatment so that when you enter a hospital, you enter a system that moves you quickly towards the next diagnosis and then the next diagnosis after that for the next component problem in a whole picture that few people will see. It's a dysfunctional system that feels like a conveyor belt. We have a disease-treatment system rather than a health-care system caring for human beings." Ms. Bennett laments, "Figuring out how much all this care during the course of an illness is almost impossible," citing that "the same CT scan in the same hospital cost $776 or $2,586, depending on which insurance company was paying." She cogently adds "We could have done better. We should all be doing better to adjust the focus on the needs of the patient, and not on the business model of the doctors, hospitals and insurance companies".

Serious gaps between health care delivery and high-quality patient-centered outcomes have been created by a lack of rigorous, systematic compliance with appropriateness criteria. As a case in point, a recent retrospective analysis from an academic medical center of a large group of CT and MRI examinations for appropriateness using evidence-based guidelines revealed that 26% did not meet appropriateness criteria [17]. In this analysis, in the appropriate study group, 58% had positive findings and affected medical management, whereas, within the inappropriate group, only 13% had positive findings and affected management. Notably, the highest percentage of inappropriate examinations was CT studies of the brain without contrast [17]. Additionally, there was a high negativity rate among these inappropriate examinations; the odds were 3.5 times higher that a negative finding would be associated with an inappropriate versus an appropriate examination. This is critical information for policy makers in the pursuit of utilization guidelines for medical imaging. Patients, physicians, payers, and the public should become better informed about the positive predictive value of imaging tests, while simultaneously making the commitment to decrease costs and ensure quality and safety in our nation's health.

A valuable resource, endorsed by the American College of Emergency Physicians to increase the appropriate use of imaging, improve quality and efficiency of emergency care, and mitigate redundant testing is health information exchange (HIE) [25]. HIE is defined as electronic sharing of health information across health care organizations within a region, community, or hospital system [26]. A recent study involving repeat emergency department (ED) patient-visits for headache (HA) is among the first to demonstrate that the use of HIE improves adherence to evidence-based guidelines, reduces avoidable CT scans, increases patient safety and improves quality of HA care [26]. However, consistent with other research, HIE showed low use rates, being accessed for repeat HA visitors only

21.9% of the time; low use being ascribed to system factors and time constraints [26, 27]. Notable in this study, more than 15% of ED visits for HA were made by repeat visitors, some of whom had as many as 46 visits to multiple EDs for HA in a 2-year period [27]. Additionally, the study documented that over two-thirds of repeat visitors to the ED for HA received a head CT [27].

The pervasive problem of low use rates in shared information technology within a community health care network was highlighted in a study published in 2012 by the University of North Carolina (UNC) School of Public Health and the Cecil G. Sheps Center for Health Services Research, exploring the common practice of repeating chest and abdominal CT imaging in caring for trauma patients transferred to Level I trauma centers [28]. The authors observed that approximately 60% of patients who had chest and abdominal scans obtained before transfer underwent repetition of one or more of these studies. The study emphasized the substantial increase of radiation exposure for the patient as well as the material increase of resource utilization and health care costs for the institution, often not reimbursed. Most importantly, perhaps, there was no difference in outcomes for patients who underwent repeat imaging. The authors affirm, "This increase in costs and risks without associated benefit is the definition of inefficient care . . . At a national level, incentives and policies to digitize all medical records by the year 2014 are in effect but compatibility of imaging systems are not explicitly included. Given that overall health care spending continues to rise at an unsustainable pace and that we rely increasingly on imaging, these systems need to be incorporated into meaningful use criteria" [28].

Toward this end, in August 2012 key requirements aimed at imaging and radiology were included in Stage 2 meaningful use requirements released in a 196-page document by the US Department of Health and Human Services (HHS). (http://www.gpo.gov/fdsys/pkg/FR-2012-09-04/pdf/2012-21050.pdf). Such requirements will serve to shape reimbursement levels from the CMS with higher incentive reimbursements going to facilities that meet the requirements and lower reimbursements for those who do not. The most important requirement calls for accessibility of imaging and radiology reports through a certified electronic health record technology (CEHRT). The HHS states that this requirement shows potential to reduce the cost and radiation exposure from imaging studies that are repeated solely due to the prior test being unavailable to the provider. In reaction to the ruling, some health care experts expressed concern over the ability of CEHRT to store images and data. HHR responded by emphasizing that CEHRT does not need to store data, it only needs to make images accessible. This aim may be readily accomplished by cloud-based image storage and retrieval from remote viewing systems. Cloud technology allows for rapid and efficient sharing of images across providers via a remote server and neutral archive, all the while providing fundamental features of data security and patient privacy [29]. Cloud technologies provide health care communities with the ability to rapidly coordinate the delivery of services using one single access point, effectively eliminating the problems of incompatibility of PACS between different hospitals, which, especially in medical emergencies, is critical for optimal care. In a pilot trial of one commercial cloud IT system in the setting of trauma patient transfer to a Level I Trauma Center, advantages of cloud IT were accentuated as it permitted preliminary imaging assessment while the patient was still en route. This enabled the trauma team to start evaluating the patient's condition and begin to coordinate care even before the patient's arrival (personal communication between D. Armao and J. Crawford and P. Petrin, Community Outreach and Informatics Specialists, School of Medicine, Department of Radiology at UNC Hospitals). Further, Stage 2 Meaningful Use calls for more than 30% of radiology orders to use computerized physician order entry (CPOE) and use of clinical decision support (CDS) software.

CT: Increasing radiation exposure versus public health and safety

A compelling body of experimental and epidemiologic evidence has linked exposure to low-dose ionizing radiation with the development of solid cancers and leukemia [30]. Over the past 30 years, the average radiation dose to which individuals in the USA are exposed has doubled [31, 32]. Although the average dose from natural background sources has remained static, the average dose from medical imaging has increased greater than sixfold [31, 32]. The biggest contributor to this dramatic increase in population medical radiation exposure is the CT scan [33]. In the USA, annual CT examinations are now approaching 80 million and increasing by approximately 10% per year [33]. The Food and Drug Administration (FDA) estimates that a CT examination with an effective dose of 10 mSv, or one CT of the abdomen, may be associated with an increased chance of developing fatal cancer for approximately one patient in 2000, whereas the Biological Effects of Ionizing Radiation (BEIR) VII lifetime risk model predicts that with the same low-dose radiation, approximately one individual in 1000 will develop cancer [30, 34]. Compared with the overall risk to the individual of developing cancer, approximately 42 per 100 individuals, imaging-based radiation risk may appear small. However, from a public health risk perspective, this small individual cancer risk must be multiplied by a large and ever-increasing population of individuals undergoing CT examinations [30, 35]. Estimates suggest that approximately 29,000 future cancers could be related to CT scan use in the USA in 2007 [36].

CT radiation doses are much higher than conventional radiography doses. For instance, one chest CT scan involves an effective dose anywhere from 100 to 1000 times greater than that from a corresponding chest X-ray (radiograph) [35]. The relatively high radiation dose of CT examinations when compared with other medical imaging studies is further compounded by the common ordering practice of multiple CT examinations on the same patient. In a large cohort, retrospective analysis spanning two decades, 33% of patients underwent five or more CT studies [37]. Such practice causes cumulative CT radiation exposure and adds incrementally to baseline cancer risk [37]. Additionally, in a recent multi-institutional analysis of radiation dose associated with common CT examinations in the San Francisco Bay Area, CA, there was substantial variation in doses within and between institutions with a 13-fold variation between the highest and lowest dose for identical CT procedures [38]. Hence, depending on where and when an individual received a CT study, the effective dose received could substantially exceed the median.

Although it is difficult to imagine modern medicine without the diagnostic strengths of CT, there is convincing evidence that a substantial fraction of the approximately 80 million annual CT exams are performed without sound medical justification. This quantitative evidence is derived from comparing actual CT use patterns with expected CT utilization if appropriate clinical decision guidelines were followed. Recent studies suggest that if appropriate clinical criteria were followed, 20–40% of CT scans could be avoided [17, 33, 39]. As a case in point, CT is commonly used to assess patients for suspected pulmonary embolism (PE). With the growing use of CT pulmonary angiography to rule out PE, it is not uncommon to include lower extremity venography to assess for deep vein thrombosis [38]. Therefore in addition to scanning the chest, the patient's pelvis and proximal thighs are imaged, thus increasing the scanning length and significantly increasing radiation exposure and cancer risk. Protocols requiring more images by increasing the scan length, which may represent scanning more anatomical regions, or repeatedly scanning through the same area (non-contrasted and contrast-enhanced scans), result in higher radiation exposure.

A landmark, recent, retrospective analysis by Mamlouk et al. of a large cohort of patients undergoing CT pulmonary angiography for possible PE showed, that in the absence of thromboembolic clinical risk factors, it is extremely unlikely (0.95% chance) to have a CT angiogram positive for PE [40]. More specifically, in this clinical setting, 90.16% of patients had a CT angiogram negative for PE, and only 6.36% patients had a CT angiogram positive for PE [40]. Such a low rate underscores the necessity and relevance for clinical risk factor evaluation prior to imaging. By contrast, analysis of risk factor assessment for PE in all patients showed a sensitivity and negative predictive value of 97.46% and 99.05 %, respectively. Importantly, addition of a relatively inexpensive, ($64.00), D-dimer test to thromboembolic risk factor assessment imparted a high sensitivity and negative predictive value of 100%, respectively. In 2008, nearly 600,000 CT pulmonary angiographic studies were performed in the USA. Charges for the studies are substantial, in the range of $3000.00 per examination [40]. Young women with associated excess estrogen state and symptoms of PE are commonly evaluated with CT angiography [41]. A recent report revealed an increased relative risk of breast and lung cancer in patients receiving one CT angiogram (estimated dose, 12–32 mSv) for PE assessment, with an especially heightened risk in younger women [41]. For breast cancer, the lifetime attributable risk (LAR) ranged from 20 excess cases per 100,000 for the PE protocol in 55-year-old women to 503 excess cases per 100,000 in 15-year-old girls [40]. Of note, in the previously cited study by Mamlouk et al., 92% of women underwent a CT angiography that was negative for PE. More recently, a large multicenter prospective study with 11 US EDs and 5940 patients enrolled reported that one-third of imaging performed for suspected PE may be categorized as avoidable [42].

Current CT imaging utilization patterns demonstrate a substantial gap between clinical indications at point-of-care versus the number of scans ordered. For instance, a retrospective analysis of trauma patients at an academic level 1 trauma center showed that application of American College of Radiology (ACR) appropriateness criteria to this cohort would have resulted in a reduction of CT exams by 44% [43]. The majority of patients were younger than 30 years at the time of imaging. Importantly, no patient with clinically significant injuries would have been excluded from CT imaging [43]. A recent, 5-year retrospective study, using National

Hospital Ambulatory Medical Care Survey (NHAMCS) data, analyzed trends in the rates of CT use and important diagnosis in ED patients with abdominal pain [44]. Several salient results were derived through this endeavor. Despite a more than doubling in CT use, there was no increase in the detection rates for appendicitis, diverticulitis, and gallbladder disease; nor was there a reduction in hospital admissions. Moreover, a study by Korley et al., comprising a 10-year retrospective analysis of use of advanced imaging for injury-related conditions in US EDs showed a threefold increase in the acquisition of CT and MRI [45]. Most notably, such a sizable increase in advanced imaging utilization occurred without a significant increase in injury-related conditions or a change in the disposition of the patient based on imaging findings. Additionally, the majority of advanced imaging examinations represented CT use. For patients who received CT or MRI, hospital visits lasted at least 2 hours longer than for those who did not receive advanced imaging. Such a swell of medical imaging rates in US EDs has numerous health policy implications, ranging from the increased cost burden that superfluous imaging exerts on the health care system to the radiation-induced oncologic risks associated with CT examinations. This latter issue is particularly pressing for younger individuals, as approximately 70% of injury-related ED visits are for those patients younger than 45 years [46]. Investigators in the study by Korley et al. asserted that additional analysis is warranted in order to understand the patient, hospital, and physician factors responsible for this increase and to optimize the risk–benefit balance of advanced radiology use. The authors concluded by stating that, "the role of evidence-adoption strategies, such as computerized decision support and audit and feedback in promoting adherence to decision rules for imaging needs to be further understood" [45].

A study by Prevedello et al. in a recent issue of *The American Journal of Medicine* [47] cited the material variation in emergency physicians' use of head CT. Study results showed that unadjusted head CT ordering rates per physician ranged from 4.4% to 16.9% overall and from 15.2% to 61.7% in adult patients diagnosed with atraumatic HA, with both rates varying significantly between physicians. Twofold variation in head CT ordering overall (6.5–13.5%) and approximately threefold variation in head CT ordering for atraumatic HA (21.2–60.1%) persisted even after controlling for pertinent variables. This pronounced variation in imaging use persisted even after controlling for factors that are known to affect imaging ordering practices. Reasons for residual variability in ordering patterns include physician knowledge gaps, practice style variation, and risk intolerance.

The authors indicted, "Quality improvement studies are needed to assess whether specific interventions, such as evidence-based computerized physician order entry (CPOE) with embedded decision support (DS) could reduce practice pattern variation by increasing the appropriateness of head CT scans ordered for patients with headache" [47].

There has been a recently approved CMS Hospital Outpatient Quality Data Reporting Program measure, which aims to assess the utility of head CTs in patients with atraumatic HA presenting to US EDs (https://www.qualitynet.org/dcs/ContentServer?c=Page&pagename=QnetPublic%2FPage%2FQnetTier3&cid=1192804531207). This measure would calculate the percentage of Medicare beneficiary patients who present with an atraumatic HA and receive a brain CT. This metric is predicated on the premise that ER physicians "may be inclined to use CT scans unnecessarily for the sake of time and caution" [48]. Driving this quality measure are the key catalysts of untenable health care cost, approximately $100 billion annually, overutilization lacking an evidence base and continuing literature on the cancer risk of ionizing radiation associated with CT examinations. Recent estimates indicate that 4000 future cancers may result from head CT examinations performed in 2007 [36].

In US EDs, the greatest increase has occurred in neuroimaging (CTs and MRIs) [49]. In a recent retrospective analysis, using the NHAMCS, in 2007, a head CT was performed in one out of every 14 ED visits, with one out of every 34 children younger than 18 years receiving a head CT [50]. Using the same NHAMCS data instrument to sharpen the focus on a more susceptible population at risk, recent research reviewing the rising use of CT in child visits to US EDs, 1995–2008, cited a fivefold increase, from 0.33 million to 1.65 million, with a compound annual growth rate of 13.2% [51]. According to Larson et al., in patients younger than 18 years, the most common complaint reported was head injury (1.94 million visits), followed by HA (1.39 million visits) and abdominal pain (0.97 million visits). Consensus statements by the ACR emphasize that the yield of positive neuroimaging studies in patients with nontraumatic HA and a normal neurologic examination is extremely low, about 0.4% and 0.9% in adults and children, respectively [52, 53]. As reflected in the former instance, 250 patients are required to undergo CT scanning in order to detect one lesion.

In 2008 the ACR joined with the Radiologic Society of North America to start the "Image Wisely" initiative, which offers education on lowering doses in all patients and ensuring appropriate test ordering [54, 55]. In April 2012, the ACR partnered with the American Board of Internal

Medicine (ABIM) Foundation's "Choosing Wisely" program, offering five tips for when *doctors and patients* should think twice before going ahead with imaging tests (Five Things Physicians and Patients Should Question www.choosingwisely.org). This reform movement was most likely inspired by medical ethicist H. Brody's landmark perspective piece, "Medicine's ethical responsibility for health care reform—The top five list," a call to arms to a profession that has sworn to put the patients' interests first [56]. According to Brody, the "top five list" would serve as a prescription for how, within a specialty, the most money could be saved most quickly without depriving any patient of meaningful medical benefit. Paramount on Brody's list "is the many common uses of CT scans, which not only add to costs but also expose patients to the risks of radiation." Most importantly, at the top of the list for the ACR/ABIM joint initiative Choosing Wisely is the injunction: Do not do imaging for uncomplicated HA.

Despite the 2010 FDA initiative to reduce unnecessary radiation exposure from medical imaging through collaboration with other federal agencies and health care professional groups, an exiguous amount of systematic, standardized, and reproducible patient education has occurred in the interim. In a recent survey by Baumann et al. involving 1168 ED patients with abdominal pain, patients were assessed as to their confidence in medical evaluations that ranged from history and physical examination only, to history and physical, laboratory testing, and CT imaging [57]. Additionally, patients were queried as to their understanding of radiation exposure and radiation-related cancer risk. The study concluded that patients reported far greater confidence in workups that included CT, yet, at the same time, substantially underestimated the radiation dose of CT relative to chest radiography. Patient comprehension of cancer risk was poor. Further, 39% of patients who reported no previous CT had, in fact, had a CT scan completed within the past 5 years, as documented in the electronic medical record (EMR). For those patients who reported a previous CT scan and had a study documented in the EMR, the mean number of scans was 5.4, with a range of 1 to 57 scans.

As the use of medical imaging continues to increase [10] and information about the health risks of ionizing radiation from imaging continues to emerge, the need for effective dialogue between health care provider and patient about the benefits and risks of such tests intensifies [58]. A study in the July issue of the *Archives of Internal Medicine* revealed that health care providers, including fourth-year medical students, attending physicians, and house staff from internal medicine, emergency medicine, radiology, cardiology, and pulmonary clinicians, infrequently educated patients about radiation risks when ordering imaging studies [59]. Specifically, of 300 respondents, 71% reported educating patients 25% of the time or less about radiation risks when ordering CT examinations. Further, 42% of providers offered that time limitations frequently prevented them from educating patients about radiation risks from medical tests and only 28% agreed that informed consent should be obtained when ordering CT exams. Interventions are warranted that will close the communication and quality improvement gap between imaging utilization and effective, open dialogue between caregiver and patient.

Especially in light of the ever-growing body of evidence that strongly implicates CT use in both ionizing radiation cancer risks and runaway health care costs, it remains to be determined whether outcomes are sufficiently improved to justify the harms and costs [60–62]. Further research on appropriate indications for neuroimaging and implementation of performance improvement programs with quality metrics that have, at their core, patient-centered care, are needed to ensure that this valuable technology is used in a safe and cost-effective fashion.

Protecting our children

The pediatric population represents a particularly vulnerable group of individuals at increased risk for cancer [63]. For example, recent risk projections suggest that for an abdominal or pelvic CT scan, the lifetime risks for children ≤15 years old are one cancer per 500 scans irrespective of age at exposure [36]. A recent keystone, large cohort retrospective analysis directly assessed the question of whether cancer risks are increased after CT scans in childhood and young adulthood, demonstrating that the use of CT scans in children to deliver cumulative doses of about 50 mGy [50 mSv) may triple the risk of leukemia, while doses of about 60 mGy [60 mSv) may triple the risk of brain cancer [60].

There exist unique considerations for radiation exposure in children, namely: 1) children are at greater risk than adults from a given dose of radiation because of enhanced radiosensitivity of developing organs [31]; 2) children have a longer life expectancy than adults and more remaining years of life during which time a radiation-induced cancer could develop [31]; 3) children may receive a higher radiation dose than necessary if CT settings are not adjusted for their smaller body size [64]; and 4) due to the surge of overutilization of medical imaging [65], individuals who are currently children are likely to eventually receive higher cumulative lifetime doses of medically related radiation than those who are currently adults [51]. A large, population-based study by Dorfman et al. showed that exposure to ionizing radiation from medical imaging may occur frequently among children [66]. Based on data gleaned from this research, the average US child in this study population will have received more than seven diagnostic imaging studies using ionizing radiation by the time he or she reaches 18 years of age. Most recently, an analysis using a robust nationally representative sample of US ED visits from 1998 to 2008 identified a steep rise in CT utilization among pediatric patients presenting with abdominal pain. In this study the authors stressed that concurrent with this overall reliance on CT imaging among young patients with abdominal pain, there was no demonstrable change in other imaging use, hospital admission, or ED diagnosis of appendicitis [67]. Despite the evidence of known cancer risks of CT related radiation, 5 to 9 million CT examinations are performed annually on children in the US (http://www.cancer.gov/cancertopics/causes/radiation/radiation-risks-pediatric-CT).

A landmark study by Larson et al. looking at nationwide trends from 1995 to 2008, cited a fivefold increase, from 0.33 million to 1.65 million, in the number of pediatric ED visits that included CT examinations [68]. Importantly, the authors noted that almost 90% of US emergency room CT scans on children was performed in non-pediatric-focused facilities. As quality performance of CT requires special oversight, especially in regard to the selection of size-based CT scanning parameters, it is possible that non-pediatric-focused radiology departments may be less likely to tailor the CT technique to the size of the pediatric patient [51]. Research looking at outside referrals from community hospitals documented that technical parameters that influence radiation dose for helical CT are not adjusted for infants, children, or adolescents, despite the tremendous variation in body size among these individuals [64]. The practice of using the same radiation exposure factors for CT examinations of children as those for adults is not uncommon [69]. Such practices in the pediatric sector result in radiation exposure that is unnecessarily and inappropriately high [64]. Evidence that the dearth of CT radiation dose reduction measures in community hospital settings continues unabated has been very recently underscored by an investigation emanating from Children's Hospital Boston and Harvard Medical School. In the setting of abdominal/pelvic CT scans for trauma performed at outside hospitals, half of the children received radiation doses exceeding the standard dose, overall ranging from 0.17 to 5.07 times [70]. On an even more troubling concluding note, the investigators asserted "Most of the CT scans failed to disclose any pathology and it may be possible that the study and its radiation risk could have been avoided entirely. A life-threatening abdominal injury is rare in hemodynamically stable children with a normal abdominal examination" [70]. There is a relative paucity of data that compare private practice, community-based and university-based practice and utilization. What may be particularly alarming, as this study infers, is that excess and inappropriate use in smaller practices with less institutional oversight is likely far worse than in major medical centers. The troubling aspect is that much of the data of overuse are derived from academic practices, which itself is very worrisome, implying that the situation may be far worse in the community setting. Rather than 30% unnecessary imaging, it may be well in excess of 50%.

In contradistinction to the community hospital setting, a recent Web-based survey which polled members of the Society for Pediatric Radiology revealed that respondents practicing in university or children's hospital settings attested to significantly decreased pediatric radiation doses for body CT [71]. The authors commented that this salutary change in pediatric CT protocols could be credited in large part to educational strategies promoted by professional societies such as the ACR practice guidelines and efforts at consciousness-raising, such as the Society of Pediatric Radiology "as low as reasonably achievable" (ALARA) concept and executive summary [72].

Despite these initiatives, marked disparity between pediatric CT scanning techniques and dose-reduction protocols in university hospital settings versus outside community hospitals and practices persists. The most urgent challenge, identified by the Alliance for Radiation Safety in Pediatric Imaging, is optimization of CT scans in children which, perforce, requires "a solid understanding of all technical aspects of CT including the most relevant scan parameters, and new dose reduction techniques" [54]. Toward this end, actionable, point-of-care, collaborative learning measures with neighboring community hospitals are warranted to close the gap between medically appropriate CT studies in children and quality health care with radiation dose reduction.

Notwithstanding ever-increasing awareness of the risks to health and safety from radiation from CT scans, Smith-Bindman, in a recent commentary published in the *Archives of Internal Medicine* exhorts "There is a pressing need for educational information for the broad medical community (i.e. not just medical physicists) to enhance understanding of the doses of radiation involved in diagnostic imaging and the health risks associated with those doses" [73].

Historical efforts to solve the problem of medical imaging overutilization: Limitations of radiology benefits management programs

Policy makers, payers, and health plans have grappled with solutions aimed at improving appropriate utilization of medical imaging. Payers have adopted methods to control utilization, with a common approach being radiology benefits management (RBM) programs. RBM programs require pre-approval before imaging studies are conducted. However, pre-authorization programs run by medical management companies and insurance companies do not provide an adequate solution. In practice, the mechanics of pre-authorization are dilatory, with significant potential to impede patient care. Further, it is not favored by the majority of physicians. RBMs fail in the real-time education of appropriateness criteria, as requests are processed by personnel in a separate area of the office, with physicians receiving little to no substantive feedback regarding their ordering requests [17]. In addition, the notion that the dramatic increase in medical imaging overutilization is solely due to the Medicare fee-for-service (FFS) population or patients with generous private insurance is spurious. Recent studies have documented overutilization of advanced imaging among HMOs [8]. Thus ever-increasing, modern imaging utilization patterns occurring in the general FFS environment pervade the managed care setting by virtue of: 1) patient care which does not consistently incorporate past medical history, signs and symptoms, and risk factor assessment in stratifying patients; 2) health-related diagnostic tests and ordering practices which are not guided by appropriateness criteria; and 3) patient expectations [8].

Prior authorization has had a long, 30-year track record in attempting to check unnecessary services by requiring authorization of a choice a clinician has already made. Despite RBM's ubiquitous presence in the US health care system as a management utilization tool, the Moran Company, engaged by the Access to Medical Imaging Coalition, stated in an executive summary that "We were unable to find a single study in the peer-reviewed health economics literature that evaluated the cost-effectiveness of prior authorization of inpatient hospital services" [74].

Notably, cost containment efforts by RBMs are generally focused on the outpatient setting, and traditionally do not target the ED. Hence, CT use, with concomitant radiation exposure and rising costs, continues unabated in the ED setting. A recently published 13-year retrospective analysis by Larson et al., using the NHAMCS database, demonstrated that the number of visits in which CT was performed in the ED increased at a compound annual growth rate of 16% [51]. The authors commented, "While the number of visits associated with CT increased nearly 600% . . . the total population radiation dose probably increased at an even higher rate." The use of CT in US EDs increased at a consistent, exponential rate, and at a higher rate than that reported in other settings [51].

The meaningful use of health information technology: Computerized decision support systems

"Medical decision support" refers to improving physician test ordering behaviors toward reducing cost, ensuring patient safety, and improving quality of care [75]. In contrast to the retrospective regulation of imaging orders after they are placed, clinical decision support tools are designed to prospectively influence the choice of tests before they are ordered. Typically, radiologists are not involved in patient care before imaging requisitions are generated. Nevertheless, the process of quality patient care in Radiology begins as early as the first physician–patient encounter. With computerized radiology order entry (ROE) and decision support (DS), physicians are asked to check off relevant indications from pre-populated lists keyed to the requested imaging examination. Indications are divided into logical groups including signs and symptoms, known diagnoses, and prior tests results, including imaging. Clicking the "submit" button serves to instantiate the imaging order. Next, immediate DS feedback is given in the form of an appropriateness score based on ACR criteria and expert specialty panel consensus.

With the consistent and standardized use of DS for imaging orders, clinicians select an intermediate to high pretest probability patient population for a study, necessarily increasing the positive predictive value of the test, meanwhile decreasing the likelihood of false-positive examinations. Hence ROE and DS mitigate the problem of overutilization of medical imaging through two important effects:
1. the direct effect of the decreased number of inappropriate imaging exams from the onset;
2. the indirect, albeit material, effect of attenuating excess health care spending, including decreased false positive examinations, that may result in re-imaging, anxiety, surgical intervention, and morbidity.

Perhaps the most critical tool for changing physician behavior is education. In the face of high patient volumes and compressed time slots for patient care, DS may offer a welcomed didactic for busy clinicians. Evidence for the strength of ROE and DS to effect a cultural change evinced through changes in ordering patterns and inappropriate use of medical imaging has been demonstrated in research from the Harvard Healthcare System, Partners Healthcare [76]. In this 7-year retrospective analysis from a large metropolitan academic medical center, substantial decreases in the growth of outpatient imaging procedures were observed coincident with the implementation of ROE and DS for referring physicians. The most impressive change occurred for CT, in which the growth rate and absolute quarterly increase, after ROE and DS system implementation, was essentially flat. Per year, the growth rates before and after ROE/DS implementation were as follows; CT 12% to 1%, and MRI 12% to 7%, respectively [76]. The authors point out that MRI volumes were affected much less than CT volumes. This effect was due to DS appropriateness feedback favoring MRI over CT for several indications, in addition to a propensity on the part of providers, abetted by concerns in the recent literature regarding radiation risks with CT scanning, to substitute MR for CT. Noteworthy in this study were contractual agreements between the large academic medical center and major regional payers to accept ROE and DS system claims without pre-authorization by RBMs. Further, an integral piece of the negotiation process was pay-for-performance incentives given to health care providers who achieved stipulated targets in reducing high-cost imaging rates.

The pervasive practice of performing excessive CT pulmonary angiography for the evaluation of PE in the ED is well established in the medical community (Chapter 2). In a very recent study by Khorasani and colleagues from the Center for Evidence Based Imaging, Brigham and Women's Hospital, implementation of evidence-based clinical decision support (CDS) in the ED was associated with a significant (20.1%) decrease in the use, as well as a significant (69.0%) increase in the yield of CT pulmonary angiography for the evaluation of acute PE in the ED during a 2-year period [77]. In this analysis, one of the most laudable aspects was the careful explanation given to the mechanics associated with the successful implementation of CDS in their health care system. This is in contrast to other hospital settings, where implementation of CDS failed to significantly decrease use of CT pulmonary angiography and led to the removal of CDS from the ED owing to noncompliance by the ED physicians [78]. In the study by Khorasani and colleagues, the authors detail: "Our roll-out strategy involved targeted general multidisciplinary discussions at faculty meetings, emergency physician champions and an education campaign around the evidence basis for our CDS strategy across our institution that, if re-enforced over time, may account for the continued reduction in use and increased yield of CT pulmonary angiography seen 2 years after implementation of CDS. We believe that all of these factors increased the acceptance of CDS implementation because a multifactorial approach to culture change has proved to be effective in other settings" [79].

Although evidence continues to emerge that CDS tools show promise in cost containment, improved health outcomes, and patient safety, diffusion of this medical imaging utilization management tool has been slow [80]. However, according to a survey conducted by the Black Book Rankings, involving 1340 clinical and information technology leaders from physician practices, hospitals, accountable care organizations (ACOs), and pharmaceutical manufacturers, 84% of health care organizations that do not have CDS plan to acquire at least one such tool within 12 months [81]. According to Black Book Rankings, only 16% of US hospitals currently have the CDS tools to manage the data needs of evolving ACOs [81].

In the wake of two decades worth of published evidence-based guidelines related to the appropriateness of ordering imaging tests, the ACR has recently contracted with the National Decision Support Company (NDSC) to render ACR appropriateness criteria the de facto CDS national standard, to be marketed as ACR Select (www.ACRSelect.org). The timing of this project is propitious, as the US Office of the National Coordinator for Health Information Technology has incorporated the use of CDS systems into meaningful use requirements [82].

Progress in reducing the overuse and misuse in imaging

In February 2010, the FDA launched an initiative to reduce unnecessary radiation from medical imaging [83]. Ultimately, the agency will mandate manufacturers to incorporate safeguards against overdosing into equipment design, require that dose information be recorded in a standard fashion for inclusion in medical records, and develop tools for patients to track their imaging history [84]. Recognizing the paramount importance of developing evidence-based criteria for appropriate imaging use in concert with standardized, diagnostic reference levels of radiation, the FDA strongly encourages professional organizations to take the initiative [84].

It is essential that physicians engage in innovative measures to improve health care delivery and contain costs. The Medicare Improvements for Patients and Providers Act (MIPPA) by the US Congress in 2008 called for accreditation of private outpatient imaging centers providing MRI, CT, PET, and nuclear medicine procedures imaging facilities by January 2012 as a condition for receiving reimbursement by Medicare for imaging services. The state of California has mandated: that the dose used for CT examinations be recorded in every patient's medical record; annual verification of each dose by a medical physicist; and the reporting of dose errors to patients, physicians, and the state [73, 85]. Spurred by the recognition of the serious potential public health risk associated with diagnostic radiation, the US Joint Commission has issued a "Sentinel Event Alert" sending an undeniable message that the possible harm of radiation exposure has come under close scrutiny [86].

A new report from the US Government Accountability Office (GAO) analyzing expenditures for advanced imaging services and self-referral from 2004 to 2010, reflects a growing commitment from national agencies to investigate ongoing sources of wasteful health care spending [87]. The report revealed that the overall incidence of self-referral increased during the period, underscoring that the number of self-referred MRI studies increased by 80% over the study period, compared with growth of 12% for non-self-referred MRI services. The GAO report added that in 2010, health care providers who self-referred likely made 400,000 more referrals for advanced imaging studies than they would have if they were not self-referring and that these superfluous self-referred studies cost Medicare $109 million. Moreover, considering that the additional referrals were unnecessary, it was correctly argued that they posed an unacceptable risk for beneficiaries, particularly in the case of CT services, which involve the use of ionizing radiation that has been linked to an increased risk of developing cancer [87].

Two important imaging synods have recently leveled congruent proactive measures in the arena of CT protocol optimization. One consortium working to mitigate CT radiation risk was sponsored by the National Institute of Biomedical Imaging and Bioengineering (NIBIB) and cosponsored by several other governmental and nongovernmental agencies involved in medical imaging [88, 89]. Many advances discussed are close to fruition, including the incorporation into CT scanner platforms of new detectors, new X-ray sources and beam filters, new imaging geometries, new approaches to data acquisition, and new iterative reconstruction methods [89]. Even with the current technology, researchers have reported substantial reductions in routine effective doses from CT compared with the National Council on Radiation Protection (NCRP) reference levels, with radiation dose reduction in children being particularly gratifying [88, 90, 91]. The second consortium represents the growing commitment by radiology practices in the USA to participate in the National CT Dose Registry sponsored by the ACR [92]. The ACR Dose Index Registry allows individual practices to monitor dose indices by comparing itself to regional and national experience and benchmark its radiation doses against similar organizations according to size and scope of procedures. The registry's long term goal is to establish national benchmarks of radiation dose reduction in ultimately developing national standards to guide improvements in the safety of CT scanning [88].

Impediments

Substantial impediments to implementation exist within the health care system. Resistance to change and medicolegal concerns are high on the list of obstacles to reform [93]. It is clear that a major driver in excessive and inappropriate utilization is medicolegal in nature, with evidence that costs of malpractice litigation are exorbitant, resulting in little practical benefit to patients or society [94]. Furthermore, with the inception of the EMR, the medicolegal implications that pertain to its employment are at present uncertain [95]. Holding medical experts accountable for their testimony and having medical experts employed as agents of the court rather than of the adversarial legal teams have been proposed as low cost means to control abuse [96]. Recently, a panel of health care experts in the NEJM proposed a strategy to reduce the costs of defensive medicine [97]. The authors promoted a promising plan that would provide a "so-called safe harbor, in which physicians would have no liability if they used qualified health-information-technology systems and adhered to evidence-based clinical practice guidelines that did not reflect defensive medicine" [97]. CDS were specified as qualified health information technology systems [97].

In order for an essential management utilization tool, such as computerized physician order entry with embedded CDS, to achieve a durable impact on health care reform, it likely must advance lock step with medicolegal reform.

Conclusions and recommendations

The story of the practice of medicine, as it has unfolded over the past two decades, is complex and often perplexing. The US health care system had, or so we thought, wrapped itself in a fine pelisse of technologic advances and specialty services, only to find within a wilderness of waste and broken communication. Somehow, through the thicket of self-interest on the part of policy makers, payers, physicians, imaging industry, and patients, there must emerge the ethical imperatives of trust and right conduct. Overutilization of medical imaging intensifies untenable costs in the US health care system and exposes individuals and the general population to unnecessary radiation doses. It is obvious that a critical part of the solution to rising health care costs and fragmentation of medical care resides in cooperation and collaboration across many sectors, including radiologists, imaging equipment industry, referring clinicians, health care service payers, and public interest groups. In keeping with honoring their patients' trust, it is appropriate that radiologists take the lead in this effort. The mantle of responsibility is on physicians' shoulders. An important focus for this work is the realignment of advanced imaging techniques with the best interests of the US public to protect and restore their health.

Considering the lack of general health care coverage of the US public, it is ironic that there exists an imbalance between those medically insured who receive too much imaging, and may either not need it and/or be harmed by it, versus those who are uninsured and do not receive necessary imaging, and are harmed by the deficiency. What is needed is thoughtful appropriate allocation of resources. To this end, in this chapter, we have championed the value of advanced computer mediated education into appropriate ordering of examinations through tools such as CDS.

Finally, radiologists need to listen to the urgent call of the IOM for a "continuously learning" health care system. As a professional community, radiologists need to accelerate integration of the best clinical knowledge into care decisions by learning where referring physicians perceive gaps in imaging guideline coverage or appropriateness criteria. Radiologists should participate in the dynamic process of continuously updating and tackling new topics that require expansion, clarification, or improvements. In the current thrust to de-emphasize the traditional, paternalistic, physician-centered health care model, radiologists should vigorously show their ability to provide a broader bandwidth of patient-centeredness by becoming true partners in the cycle of care of every patient.

References

1. PricewaterhouseCoopers' Health Research Institute. The price of excess: Identifying waste in healthcare spending. Available online at: http://pwchealth.com/cgi-local/hregister.cgi/reg/waste.pdf. [accessed February 28, 2013].

2. OECD Public Affairs Division, Public Affairs and Communications Directorate. OECD Annual Report 2005; 143. Available online at: http://www.oecd.org/about/34711139.pdf. [accessed February 28, 2013].

3. Fineberg HV. Shattuck Lecture. A successful and sustainable health system—how to get there from here. N Engl J Med 2012; 366:1020–1027.

4. Redberg RF. Getting to best care at lower cost. JAMA Intern Med 2013; 173:91–92.

5. Institute of Medicine of the National Academies. Best care at lower cost: The path to continuously learning health care in America. 2012. Available online at: http://books.nap.edu/openbook.php?record_id=13444&page=R1. [accessed on February 28, 2013].

6. Amis ES, Jr., Butler PF, Applegate KE, et al. American College of Radiology white paper on radiation dose in medicine. J Am Coll Radiol 2007; 4:272–284.

7. Medicare Payment Advisory Commission. A Data Book: Healthcare Spending and the Medicare Program, June 2012. Available online at: http://www.medpac.gov/documents/Jun12DataBookEntireReport.pdf. [accessed on March 6, 2013].

8. Smith-Bindman R, Miglioretti DL, Larson EB. Rising use of diagnostic medical imaging in a large integrated health system. Health Aff (Millwood) 2008; 27:1491–1502.

9. Dinan MA, Curtis LH, Hammill BG, et al. Changes in the use and costs of diagnostic imaging among Medicare beneficiaries with cancer, 1999–2006. JAMA 2010; 303:1625–1631.

10. Smith-Bindman R, Miglioretti DL, Johnson E, et al. Use of diagnostic imaging studies and associated radiation exposure for patients enrolled in large integrated health care systems, 1996–2010. JAMA 2012; 307:2400–2409.

11. Hendee WR, Becker GJ, Borgstede JP, et al. Addressing overutilization in medical imaging. Radiology 2010; 257:240–245.

12. Iglehart JK. Health insurers and medical-imaging policy—a work in progress. N Engl J Med 2009; 360:1030–1037.

13. Fisher ES, Wennberg DE, Stukel TA, et al. The implications of regional variations in Medicare spending. Part 1: The content, quality, and accessibility of care. Ann Intern Med 2003; 138:273–287.

14. Fisher ES, Wennberg DE, Stukel TA, et al. The implications of regional variations in Medicare spending. Part 2: Health outcomes and satisfaction with care. Ann Intern Med 2003; 138:288–298.

15. Dunnick NR, Applegate KE, Arenson RL. The inappropriate use of imaging studies: A report of the 2004 Intersociety Conference. J Am Coll Radiol 2005; 2:401–406.

16. Aaron HJ. Waste, we know you are out there. N Engl J Med 2008; 359: 1865–1867.

17. Lehnert BE, Bree RL. Analysis of appropriateness of outpatient CT and MRI referred from primary care clinics at an academic medical center: How critical is the need for improved decision support? J Am Coll Radiol 2010; 7:192–197.

18. Swensen SJ. Patient-centered imaging. Am J Med 2012; 125:115–117.

19. Miller RA, Sampson NR, Flynn JM. The prevalence of defensive orthopaedic imaging: A prospective practice audit in Pennsylvania. J Bone Joint Surg Am 2012; 94:e18.

20. Yasaitis L, Fisher ES, Skinner JS, et al. Hospital quality and intensity of spending: Is there an association? Health Aff (Millwood) 2009; 28:w566–572.

21. Hu YY, Kwok AC, Jiang W, et al. High-cost imaging in elderly patients with stage IV cancer. J Natl Cancer Inst 2012; 104:1164–1172.

22. NCCN Clinical Practice Guidelines in Oncology: Colon Cancer. Available online at: http://www.nccn.org/professionals/physician_gls/f_guidelines.asp#site and also at: http://www.nccn.org/patients/patient_guidelines/colon/index.html [accessed on March 6, 2013].

23. Yabroff KR, Warren JL. High-cost imaging in elderly patients with stage IV cancer: Challenges for research, policy, and practice. J Natl Cancer Inst 2012; 104:1113–1114.

24. Bennett A. Why did her husband's end-of-life care cost so much? In: Newsweek, May 28th, 2012.

25. American College of Emergency Physicians. Health information technology. Ann Emerg Med 2008; 52:595.

26. Bailey JE, Wan JY, Mabry LM, et al. Does health information exchange reduce unnecessary neuroimaging and improve quality of headache care in the emergency department? J Gen Intern Med 2012.

27. Vest JR, Zhao H, Jasperson J, et al. Factors motivating and affecting health information exchange usage. J Am Med Inform Assoc 2011; 18:143–149.

28. Emick DM, Carey TS, Charles AG, et al. Repeat imaging in trauma transfers: A retrospective analysis of computed tomography scans repeated upon arrival to a Level I trauma center. J Trauma Acute Care Surg 2012; 72:1255–1262.

29. Roney K. 6 valuable outcomes cloud technologies offer hospitals. In: Becker's Hospital Review—Business & legal issues for health system leadership 2012. Available online at: http://www.beckershospitalreview.com/healthcare-information-technology/6-valuable-outcomes-cloud-technologies-offer-hospitals.html. [accessed on February 28, 2013].

30. Committee to Assess Health Risks from Exposure to Low Levels of Ionizing Radiation, National Research Council. Executive Summary. In: Board on Radiation Effects Research—Division on Earth and Life Studies, ed. Health Risks from Exposure to Low Levels of Ionizing Radiation: BEIR VII – Phase 2. Washington, D.C.: The National Academies Press, 2005.

31. Brenner DJ, Hall EJ. Computed tomography—an increasing source of radiation exposure. N Engl J Med 2007; 357:2277–2284.

32. Mettler FA, Jr., Bhargavan M, Faulkner K, et al. Radiologic and nuclear medicine studies in the United States and worldwide: Frequency, radiation dose, and comparison with other radiation sources—1950–2007. Radiology 2009; 253:520–531.

33. Brenner DJ, Hricak H. Radiation exposure from medical imaging: Time to regulate? JAMA 2010; 304:208–209.

34. FDA. What are the Radiation Risks from CT? U.S. Food and Drug Administration 2005. Available online at: http://www.fda.gov/ForConsumers/ConsumerUpdates/ucm115329.htm. [accessed on March 6, 2013].

35. Semelka RC, Armao DM, Elias J, Jr., et al. Imaging strategies to reduce the risk of radiation in CT studies, including selective substitution with MRI. J Magn Reson Imaging 2007; 25:900–909.

36. Berrington de Gonzalez A, Mahesh M, Kim KP, et al. Projected cancer risks from computed tomographic scans performed in the United States in 2007. Arch Intern Med 2009; 169:2071–2077.

37. Sodickson A, Baeyens PF, Andriole KP, et al. Recurrent CT, cumulative radiation exposure, and associated radiation-induced cancer risks from CT of adults. Radiology 2009; 251:175–184.

38. Smith-Bindman R, Lipson J, Marcus R, et al. Radiation dose associated with common computed tomography examinations and the associated lifetime attributable risk of cancer. Arch Intern Med 2009; 169:2078–2086.

39. Kuppermann N, Holmes JF, Dayan PS, et al. Identification of children at very low risk of clinically-important brain injuries after head trauma: A prospective cohort study. Lancet 2009; 374:1160–1170.

40. Mamlouk MD, vanSonnenberg E, Gosalia R, et al. Pulmonary embolism at CT angiography: Implications for appropriateness, cost, and radiation exposure in 2003 patients. Radiology 2010; 256:625–632.

41. Hurwitz LM, Reiman RE, Yoshizumi TT, et al. Radiation dose from contemporary cardiothoracic multidetector CT protocols with an anthropomorphic female phantom: Implications for cancer induction. Radiology 2007; 245:742–750.

42. Venkatesh AK, Kline JA, Courtney DM, et al. Evaluation of pulmonary embolism in the emergency department and consistency with a national quality measure: Quantifying the opportunity for improvement. Arch Intern Med 2012; 172:1028–1032.

43. Hadley JL, Agola J, Wong P. Potential impact of the American College of Radiology appropriateness criteria on CT for trauma. AJR Am J Roentgenol 2006; 186:937–942.

44. Pines JM. Trends in the rates of radiography use and important diagnoses in emergency department patients with abdominal pain. Med Care 2009; 47:782–786.

45. Korley FK, Pham JC, Kirsch TD. Use of advanced radiology during visits to US emergency departments for injury-related conditions, 1998–2007. JAMA 2010; 304:1465–1471.

46. Pitts SR, Niska RW, Xu J, et al. National Hospital Ambulatory Medical Care Survey: 2006 emergency department summary. Natl Health Stat Report 2008:1–38.

47. Prevedello LM, Raja AS, Zane RD, et al. Variation in use of head computed tomography by emergency physicians. Am J Med 2012; 125:356–364.

48. Barrett TW, Schriger DL. Annals of Emergency Medicine Journal Club. Computed tomography imaging in the emergency department: Benefits, risks and risk ratios. Ann Emerg Med 2011; 58:463–464.

49. Andruchow JE, Raja AS, Prevedello LM, et al. Variation in head computed tomography use for emergency department trauma patients and physician risk tolerance. Arch Intern Med 2012; 172:660–661.

50. Raja AS, Andruchow J, Zane R, et al. Use of neuroimaging in US emergency departments. Arch Intern Med 2011; 171:260–262.

51. Larson DB, Johnson LW, Schnell BM, et al. National trends in CT use in the emergency department: 1995–2007. Radiology 2011; 258:164–173.

52. Hayes LL, Coley BD, Karmazyn B, et al. Headache—Child. ACR Appropriateness Criteria®. American College of Radiology 2012. Available online at: http://www.acr.org/~/media/ACR/Documents/AppCriteria/Diagnostic/HeadacheChild.pdf [accessed on March 6, 2013].

53. Jordan JE, Wippold II FJ, Cornelius RS, et al. Headache. ACR Appropriateness Criteria®. American College of Radiology 2009. Available online at: http://www.acr.org/~/media/ACR/Documents/AppCriteria/Diagnostic/Headache.pdf [accessed on March 6, 2013].

54. Goske MJ, Applegate KE, Bulas D, et al. Image Gently: Progress and challenges in CT education and advocacy. Pediatr Radiol 2011; 41 Suppl 2:461–466.

55. Goske MJ, Applegate KE, Boylan J, et al. The 'Image Gently' campaign: Increasing CT radiation dose awareness through a national education and awareness program. Pediatr Radiol 2008; 38:265–269.

56. Brody H. Medicine's ethical responsibility for health care reform—the Top Five list. N Engl J Med 2010; 362:283–285.

57. Baumann BM, Chen EH, Mills AM, et al. Patient perceptions of computed tomographic imaging and their understanding of radiation risk and exposure. Ann Emerg Med 2011; 58:1–7 e2.

58. Semelka RC, Armao DM, Elias J, Jr., et al. The information imperative: Is it time for an informed consent process explaining the risks of medical radiation? Radiology 2012; 262:15–18.

59. Stickrath C, Druck J, Hensley N, et al. Patient and health care provider discussions about the risks of medical imaging: not ready for prime time. Arch Intern Med 2012; 172:1037–1038.

60. Pearce MS, Salotti JA, Little MP, et al. Radiation exposure from CT scans in childhood and subsequent risk of leukaemia and brain tumours: A retrospective cohort study. Lancet 2012; 380:499–505.

61. Kocher KE, Meurer WJ, Fazel R, et al. National trends in use of computed tomography in the emergency department. Ann Emerg Med 2011; 58:452–462 e453.

62. Lateef TM, Grewal M, McClintock W, et al. Headache in young children in the emergency department: Use of computed tomography. Pediatrics 2009; 124: e12–17.

63. Dixon AK, Dendy P. Spiral CT: How much does radiation dose matter? Lancet 1998; 352:1082–1083.

64. Paterson A, Frush DP, Donnelly LF. Helical CT of the body: Are settings adjusted for pediatric patients? AJR Am J Roentgenol 2001; 176:297–301.

65. Armao D, Semelka RC, Elias J, Jr. Radiology's ethical responsibility for healthcare reform: Tempering the overutilization of medical imaging and trimming down a heavyweight. J Magn Reson Imaging 2012; 35:512–517.

66. Dorfman AL, Fazel R, Einstein AJ, et al. Use of medical imaging procedures with ionizing radiation in children: A population-based study. Arch Pediatr Adolesc Med 2011; 165:458–464.

67. Fahimi J, Herring A, Harries A, et al. Computed tomography use among children presenting to emergency departments with abdominal pain. Pediatrics 2012; 130:e1069–e1075.

68. Larson DB, Johnson LW, Schnell BM, et al. Rising use of CT in child visits to the emergency department in the United States, 1995–2008. Radiology 2011; 259:793–801.

69. Rogers LF. Taking care of children: Check out the parameters used for helical CT. AJR Am J Roentgenol 2001; 176:287.

70. Calvert C, Strauss KJ, Mooney DP. Variation in computed tomography radiation dose in community hospitals. J Pediatr Surg 2012; 47:1167–1169.

71. Arch ME, Frush DP. Pediatric body MDCT: A 5-year follow-up survey of scanning parameters used by pediatric radiologists. AJR Am J Roentgenol 2008; 191:611–617.

72. Slovis TL. The ALARA concept in pediatric CT: Myth or reality? Radiology 2002; 223:5–6.

73. Smith-Bindman R. Environmental causes of breast cancer and radiation from medical imaging: findings from the Institute of Medicine report. Arch Intern Med 2012; 172:1023–1027.

74. The Moran Company. Executive Summary. Assessing the Budgetary Implications of Alternative Strategies to Influence Utilization of Diagnostic Imaging Services 2011. Available online at: http://rightscanrighttime.org/wp-content/uploads/2011/10/AMIC-Final-UM-Report-101820114.pdf. [accessed on February 28, 2013].

75. Khorasani R. Computerized physician order entry and decision support: Improving the quality of care. Radiographics 2001; 21:1015–1018.

76. Sistrom CL, Dang PA, Weilburg JB, et al. Effect of computerized order entry with integrated decision support on the growth of outpatient procedure volumes: Seven-year time series analysis. Radiology 2009; 251:147–155.

77. Raja AS, Ip IK, Prevedello LM, et al. Effect of computerized clinical decision support on the use and yield of CT pulmonary angiography in the emergency department. Radiology 2012; 262:468–474.

78. Drescher FS, Chandrika S, Weir ID, et al. Effectiveness and acceptability of a computerized decision support system using modified Wells criteria for evaluation of suspected pulmonary embolism. Ann Emerg Med 2011; 57:613–621.

79. Schein EH. Organizational Culture and Leadership. New York, NY: John Wiley & Sons, Inc., 2010.

80. Duszak R, Jr., Berlin JW. Utilization management in radiology, Part 1: Rationale, history, and current status. J Am Coll Radiol 2012; 9:694–699.

81. American Medical Association. Health organizations express need for clinical decision support tools. News in brief—Aug. 13, 2012. Available online at: http://www.ama-assn.org/amednews/2012/08/13/bibf0813.htm. [accessed on February 28, 2013]

82. Fornell D. Government releases Stage 2 Meaningful Use Final Rule. Imaging Technology News, 2012. Available online at: http://www.itnonline.com/article/government-releases-stage-2-meaningful-use-final-rule [accessed on February 28, 2013].

83. FDA. Initiative to reduce unnecessary radiation exposure from medical imaging. Available online at: http://www.fda.gov/Radiation-EmittingProducts/RadiationSafety/RadiationDoseReduction/default.htm. [accessed on February 28, 2013].

84. Smith-Bindman R. Is computed tomography safe? N Engl J Med 2010; 363:1–4.
85. Bill SB 1237. Radiation control: Health facilities and clinics: Records. Available online at: http://www.leginfo.ca.gov/pub/09-10/bill/sen/sb_1201-1250/sb_1237_bill_20100902_enrolled.html. [accessed on February 28, 2013].
86. The Joint Comission. Sentinel Event Alert: Radiation risks of diagnostic imaging 2011. Available online at: http://www.jointcommission.org/assets/1/18/sea_471.pdf. [accessed on February 28, 2013].
87. GAO. Medicare. Higher use of advanced imaging services by providers who self-refer costing Medicare millions. United States Government Accountability Office (GAO). Report to Congressional Requesters 2012; 52. Available online at: http://www.gao.gov/assets/650/648988.pdf. [accessed on February 28, 2013].
88. Thrall JH. Radiation exposure in CT scanning and risk: Where are we? Radiology 2012; 264:325–328.
89. McCollough CH, Chen GH, Kalender W, et al. Achieving routine submillisievert CT scanning: Report from the summit on management of radiation dose in CT. Radiology 2012; 264:567–580.
90. Borgen L, Kalra MK, Laerum F, et al. Application of adaptive non-linear 2D and 3D postprocessing filters for reduced dose abdominal CT. Acta Radiol 2012; 53: 335–342.
91. Singh S, Kalra MK, Shenoy-Bhangle AS, et al. Radiation dose reduction with hybrid iterative reconstruction for pediatric CT. Radiology 2012; 263:537–546.
92. Morin RL, Coombs LP, Chatfield MB. ACR Dose Index Registry. J Am Coll Radiol 2011; 8:288–291.
93. Ryan AF, Semelka RC, Molina PL, et al. Evaluation of radiologist interpretive performance using blinded reads by multiple external readers. Invest Radiol 2010; 45:211–216.
94. Studdert DM, Mello MM, Gawande AA, et al. Claims, errors, and compensation payments in medical malpractice litigation. N Engl J Med 2006; 354:2024–2033.
95. Mangalmurti SS, Murtagh L, Mello MM. Medical malpractice liability in the age of electronic health records. N Engl J Med 2010; 363:2060–2067.
96. Semelka RC. Reply. AJR Am J Roentgenol 2011; 196:W490–W491.
97. Emanuel E, Tanden N, Altman S, et al. A systemic approach to containing health care spending. N Engl J Med 2012; 367:949–954.

CHAPTER 7

Radiology medical education

Jorge Elias Jr[1] and Richard C. Semelka[2]
[1] The School of Medicine of Ribeirao Preto, University of Sao Paulo, Brazil
[2] University of North Carolina at Chapel Hill, School of Medicine, Department of Radiology, Chapel Hill, NC, USA

The US health care system has done an excellent job at standardization of training and the use of formal examinations to ensure that physicians are well trained. Some of the other developed nations have succeeded by emulating the US system. Remarkably, however, many developed nations do not have a formalized curriculum and final examination after training. In the USA, the specialty of Radiology has been the only accredited specialty to have final exams administered during the course of the training period. Beginning in 2013, the new Radiology final board examination will be taken approximately 15 months following completion of the 4-year Radiology residency training program.

Scope of the issue

Radiology, as a medical specialty, is facing a new demand from both patients and referring clinicians for high-quality, skilled, subspecialized expertise and diagnostic certainty [1]. So far, training, certifying, and maintaining the certification have been the basis of a successful formula to keep medical specialty education, including Radiology, at a high standard in the USA. The American Board of Radiology (ABR), formed in 1934, has been the overseeing body for certification in diagnostic radiology. Seeking to keep pace with changes in medicine as a whole, in 2007 the ABR announced new requirements and testing for the board examinations, which will take full effect in 2015 [2].

Health Care Reform in Radiology, First Edition. Richard C. Semelka and Jorge Elias Jr.
© 2013 John Wiley & Sons, Inc. Published 2013 by John Wiley & Sons, Inc.

ABR certification in diagnostic radiology currently consists of three examinations: 1) a qualifying ("physics") written examination in radiologic physics that can be taken during the second or later years of training; 2) a qualifying ("written") examination in diagnostic radiology—also known as "the clinical examination"—taken in the third or fourth year of training; and 3) an oral certifying examination that covers 11 subspecialties of diagnostic radiology, each of which must be passed [2]. The certifying examination is taken near the end of the final residency year [2]. The new changes will create only two examinations. The first will be a "core examination" given at the end of the third year of radiology training (36 months; end of postgraduate year 4). The core examination will include segments on all 11 clinical categories, including basic and clinically applied physics. The core examination will include case-based material and, unlike the current qualifying examinations, will be image-rich. Fifteen months after residency there will be a computer-based certifying examination bearing structural similarity to the examinations to be administered once in each maintenance of certification (MOC) cycle throughout the diplomate's career [2]. Although changes to conform with modernization were needed, these changes have raised concerns in the radiology community [3–5]. Most of the expressed concerns relate to the impact that changes will create in the crystallized state of the established format of residency programs throughout the country (i.e. the fear of the new and the pros and cons of interested parties). Perhaps the discussion should be focused on how these changes will affect the curriculum and how to deal with the tremendous amount of knowledge that each resident in training has to assimilate. Competency evaluations during the training years are also a subject of discussion, and some authors have opined that these interim evaluations, using a consistent structure, may be an effective tool to ascertain that the Radiology residents are gleaning the required information during the course of their residency [6]. This one report studying the implementation of end-of-rotation examinations concluded that they are relatively straightforward to implement and facilitate recurring, structured, and meaningful resident evaluation and feedback [6].

While discussing trends in radiology training, McLoud states that the focus must be directed to four components related to training in radiology: 1) the selection process of new trainees; 2) the development of a standardized curriculum; 3) the protection and enhancement of research training and the creation of certification; and 4) the maintenance of certification standards [1]. In fact, the perception of the specialty of Radiology by medical school graduates has changed over recent years, which may be reflected by the shortage of radiologists in the beginning of the last decade [7]. Much of that can be explained by the steady increase of the workload of radiologists without the corresponding compensation [8], although there is evidence to suggest that a surplus of at least 3% has been reached between 2003 and 2007 [9].

Maintenance of certification and self-assessment modules

Graduates from Radiology programs since 2001 have the requirement of undergoing recertification every 10 years [10]. This requirement is not necessary for graduates from earlier years, although they are still allowed, perhaps encouraged, to undergo this same process [10]. In this recertification process radiologists can request to undergo examination in their preferred field (e.g. Neuroradiology).

The Accreditation Council for Graduate Medical Education (ACGME) has established six competencies for residency training programs, which are intrinsically present in the components of the MOC:

1. Patient care;
2. Medical knowledge;
3. Practice-based learning and improvement;
4. Interpersonal and communication skills;
5. Professionalism;
6. Systems-based practice.

Maintenance of state licensure is also a necessary requirement for a radiologist to practice. This is generally achieved by obtaining a certain number of continuing medical education (CME) credits throughout the course of the year. Maintenance of CME requirements is generally important to maintain licensure in the particular state where the radiologist practices. The four parts of the MOC [11] are:

- **Part I Professional standing**: Continuous possession of an unrestricted medical license;
- **Part II: Lifelong learning**: 25 CME credits and two self-assessment modules (SAMS) per year over the 10-year cycle;
- **Part III Cognitive examination**: Taken during years 7–10 of the cycle, this examination is based on the practice profile of the radiologist and includes four clinical modules and one general content (patient safety, contrast reactions, ethics, and so forth) module;
- **Part IV Practice quality improvement**: Radiologists must show continuous involvement in individual-, institutional-, or society-based quality improvement projects.

The ABR sets the standard lengths of training for each subspecialty during the course of the residency program, which is standardized throughout the USA.

Future directions

A future addition to the SAMS program for MOC as a radiologist in the USA relates to the issue discussed in the chapter on medicolegal reform (Chapter 9). Our opinion is that medical experts of all types—therefore including radiologists—in the ideal situation should act as agents of the court rather than partisan agents of adversarial legal teams. The partisan arrangement lends itself, perhaps elicits, unethical behavior as far as presentation of material is directed toward supporting one or other cause, rather than the truth. This makes it especially problematic to try cases "fairly," as medical information is sufficiently complex in the modern age; it is difficult enough for physicians in different specialties/subspecialties to understand or appreciate the subtleties of specialized medical care, let alone members of the general public. In our construct, radiologists would sign up to be part of a large pool of potential medical experts, acting on the part of the court, and for the act of enlisting they receive a certain amount of SAMS—perhaps 5. Then for every case they handle they receive an additional 5 points. In fact this approach to CME and SAMS may more closely reflect what is intended with these programs, which is evidence of ongoing learning to keep one competent in one's field, by emulating, in an interrogatable fashion, true radiology practice. The reads would be blinded reads, where the reviewer is provided with only the information of the interpreting radiologist received. This may be the best manner to ensure that justice is truly blind for all concerned parties, including the patient. It would be optional whether the reviewer would receive comparison data to other blinded reviewers in the case (we would recommend three to four reviewers per case); this could then be used as a grading system either simply for self-improvement or also as a means of testing a radiologist's ability for MOC. In fact, this form of follow-up information is already provided by many journals (e.g. *Radiology*), and as a reviewer one can see not only one's own review, but the reviews of the other reviewers, and the final decision. Our recommendation is essentially the same concept but used in the setting of interpreting radiology studies blindly. We would recommend using a comparison approach, which we have previously reported on, in which each described finding must get an

80% description rate (that is 80% of the reviewing radiologists made that finding) in order to be interpreted as "real." A fuller description can be found in the publication "Evaluation of radiologist interpretive performance using blinded reads by multiple external readers" by Ryan et al., 2010 [12].

Radiology education beyond Radiology residency—medical students and residents from other areas

Although residency is considered to be indispensable for consolidating knowledge of radiology, it is essential to any medical school to have radiology teaching included in the curricula [13]. In 1994 du Cret et al. reported that the overwhelming majority of clinicians in all specialties believed that formal radiologic instruction should be mandatory for medical students [13]. Imaging interpretation was believed to be an indispensable part of a medical student radiology rotation, but many clinicians indicated a need for additional training. A marked disparity in the perceived level of confidence in interpreting radiologic tests during medical school and residency between those who had and those who had not received formal radiologic instruction during medical school was evident. The authors noted that this difference in perceived level of confidence was present even among the most experienced clinicians [13].

Diagnostic imaging training begins during medical school years, although the content amount and intensity of training experience can vary widely at various institutions. Even so, competency in basic radiology skills is not an easy goal for medical education. Marchiori et al. showed that students demonstrated poor ability to recognize, categorize, manage, and identify common radiographic pathologic conditions when facing two different examination tests [14]. They also stated that educators cannot rely on National Board scores and course grades to determine student clinical competency [14]. Although their results should cause some concern for educators who use content-based radiology curricula, the authors concluded that in order to fix the problem, more radiology clinical competency exercises that emphasize film interpretation need to be incorporated into content-based curricula [14].

In the age of informatics and the Internet it is relatively clear that radiology education should be built in a fashion that simulates the actual manipulation of software and computer tools used by radiologists during case interpretation in order to motivate and improve content retention by medical students. It is a daunting task, but there is solid evidence that this strategy is worthwhile [15–17]. Most medical students prefer to learn radiology in an active context [18]. They prefer being given adequate time to find abnormalities on images, with feedback afterward from instructors [18]. Medical students prefer to be asked questions in a way that is constructive and not belittling, to realize their knowledge deficits, and to have daily expectation to come prepared [18].

When medical education comes to the expected knowledge about risks of medical radiation it is clear that much needs to be done. There is worldwide experience that even practicing physicians show lack of awareness regarding ionizing radiation hazards [19–24]. Not surprisingly, the same occurs among senior medical students and interns [25, 26]. Those evidences highlight the urgent need for improved education to minimize unnecessary exposure of patients and the community to radiation.

Referring physicians from all specialties have been challenged by the fast pace of change in diagnostic imaging, encompassing new applications and multiplicity of techniques and protocols for all modalities. CME has an essential role in keeping physician knowledge current. Nonetheless, to construct programs and confirm positive evidence takes time and financial resources.

Conclusions

It is beyond question that the structured and well-organized curriculum of Radiology residency programs in the USA, including an emphasis on research, is unsurpassed elsewhere in the world. The US educational system has served as the model for the most progressive of developed nations and should continue to do so for many years to come. It is important to keep pressing for a unified content of radiology training in medical schools worldwide, which should include minimal radiology competency and knowledge of patient safety regarding radiation hazards and other radiological safety issues.

References

1. McLoud TC. Trends in radiologic training: National and international implications. Radiology 2010; 256:343–347.
2. Alderson PO, Becker GJ. The new requirements and testing for American Board of Radiology certification in diagnostic radiology. Radiology 2008; 248:707–709.

3. Hall FM, Janower ML. The new requirements and testing for American Board of Radiology certification: A contrary opinion. Radiology 2008; 248:710–712.
4. Ruchman RB, Kwak AJ, Jaeger J. The written clinical diagnosis board examination: Survey of program director and resident opinions. AJR Am J Roentgenol 2008; 191:954–961.
5. Larson DB, Saket DD. My old Kentucky home, goodnight: Potential impact of planned changes in the radiology board certification process. AJR Am J Roentgenol 2008; 190:1149–1151.
6. Phelps A, Naeger DM, MacKenzie J, et al. Educating radiology residents in the new era: Implementation and evaluation of online end-of-rotation examinations. Acad Radiol 2011; 18:1442–1446.
7. Maynard CD. Radiology: Future challenges. Radiology 2001; 219:309–312.
8. Bhargavan M, Sunshine JH. Workload of radiologists in the United States in 2002–2003 and trends since 1991–1992. Radiology 2005; 236:920–931.
9. Soni K, Bhargavan M, Forman HP, et al. Who's underworked and who's overworked now? An update on radiologist shortage and surplus. AJR Am J Roentgenol 2010; 194:697–703.
10. Berquist TH. Maintenance of certification: Everyone needs to participate. AJR Am J Roentgenol 2008; 191:635–636.
11. Strife JL, Kun LE, Becker GJ, et al. The American board of radiology perspective on maintenance of certification: Part IV—practice quality improvement for diagnostic radiology. Radiology 2007; 243:309–313.
12. Ryan AF, Semelka RC, Molina PL, et al. Evaluation of radiologist interpretive performance using blinded reads by multiple external readers. Invest Radiol 2010; 45:211–216.
13. du Cret RP, Weinberg EJ, Sellers TA, et al. Role of radiology in medical education: Perspective of nonradiologists. Acad Radiol 1994; 1:70–74.
14. Marchiori DM, Henderson CN, Adams TL. Developing a clinical competency examination in radiology: Part II—test results. J Manipulative Physiol Ther 1999; 22:63–74.
15. Foran DJ, Nosher JL, Siegel R, et al. Dynamic quiz bank: A portable tool set for authoring and managing distributed, Web-based educational programs in radiology. Acad Radiol 2003; 10:52–57.
16. Grunewald M, Heckemann RA, Gebhard H, et al. COMPARE radiology: Creating an interactive Web-based training program for radiology with multimedia authoring software. Acad Radiol 2003; 10:543–553.
17. Chew FS, Ochoa ER, Jr., Relyea-Chew A. Application of the case method in medical student radiology education. Acad Radiol 2005; 12:746–751.
18. Zou L, King A, Soman S, et al. Medical students' preferences in radiology education a comparison between the Socratic and didactic methods utilizing powerpoint features in radiology education. Acad Radiol 2011; 18:253–256.
19. Bury B. Doctors' knowledge of exposure to ionising radiation: Finding was not surprising. BMJ 2003; 327:1166.
20. Correia MJ, Hellies A, Andreassi MG, et al. Lack of radiological awareness among physicians working in a tertiary-care cardiological centre. Int J Cardiol 2005; 103:307–311.

21. Finestone A, Schlesinger T, Amir H, et al. Do physicians correctly estimate radiation risks from medical imaging? Arch Environ Health 2003; 58:59–61.

22. Lee CI, Haims AH, Monico EP, et al. Diagnostic CT scans: Assessment of patient, physician, and radiologist awareness of radiation dose and possible risks. Radiology 2004; 231:393–398.

23. Rahman N, Dhakam S, Shafqut A, et al. Knowledge and practice of radiation safety among invasive cardiologists. J Pak Med Assoc 2008; 58:119–122.

24. Shiralkar S, Rennie A, Snow M, et al. Doctors' knowledge of radiation exposure: Questionnaire study. BMJ 2003; 327:371–372.

25. Hagi SK, Khafaji MA. Medical students' knowledge of ionizing radiation and radiation protection. Saudi Med J 2011; 32:520–524.

26. Arslanoglu A, Bilgin S, Kubal Z, et al. Doctors' and intern doctors' knowledge about patients' ionizing radiation exposure doses during common radiological examinations. Diagn Interv Radiol 2007; 13:53–55.

CHAPTER 8

Quality metrics for radiology practice

Richard C. Semelka[1] and Jorge Elias Jr[2]

[1] University of North Carolina at Chapel Hill, School of Medicine, Department of Radiology, Chapel Hill, NC, USA
[2] The School of Medicine of Ribeirao Preto, University of Sao Paulo, Brazil

Much effort has been directed to assess quality of radiology practice. Particular emphasis on quality and safety as a distinct mission in Radiology has been formalized over the last 5 years. In this chapter we present a succinct, simplified overview of the essential components to a quality program. The two main elements are the quality of the studies performed and the quality of the interpretation. Quality of imaging studies has been long described as Quality Assurance (QA). With digital imaging in the current era it is relatively straightforward to deliver a quality product. Attention has to be made, though, to safety aspects: this includes that the studies are appropriately coned down (especially in pediatrics) and that only sufficient kilovolts peak (kVp) and milliamp seconds (mAs) are delivered to result in a diagnostically accurate study. As coning can be achieved in post-processing, and administering higher radiation doses in CT does not reflect itself in the images, it is imperative that considerable effort is directed to train technologists not to take shortcuts that can result in higher radiation doses to patients.

Our intention in this chapter is not to present a comprehensive in-depth treatment of this subject but rather to present key components to a quality program. In particular we emphasize a novel strategy that targets the core of a quality program, assessment of the quality of radiological interpretation, and we perform this by using an anonymous survey directed to the customer base. This will be described herein.

Health Care Reform in Radiology, First Edition. Richard C. Semelka and Jorge Elias Jr.
© 2013 John Wiley & Sons, Inc. Published 2013 by John Wiley & Sons, Inc.

Overview

In this chapter we will describe our experience with a developed and implemented set of quality and safety programs. This is an abbreviated program compared with that described in the literature by authorities on this subject, who emphasize principles that have been termed key performance indicators (KPIs) [1, 2]. However we emphasize what we consider the most important aspect of quality assessment, which other programs gloss over: the determination of performance of the radiologists themselves, and not tangential surrogates.

The guiding principle in our programs has been to develop initiatives that: 1) are fundamentally objective and quantitative, and 2) address critical issues in Radiology practice. The concept of rendering the data quantitative is that it allows for the establishment of objective goals and standards that members of the faculty of the Department of Radiology can use to gauge their status and serve as a nonconfrontational guide for their improvement. This also provides metrics for the department to evaluate the current standard of performance and to measure progress. As an example, we will illustrate our own evolution in thought into further expansion of existing programs and development of new programs that are planned for the near future. In centers that do not have a well-developed quality program, we hope that we can provide guidance to develop a straightforward quality program that does not add tremendous complexity to function in the department, while still addressing the critical issues.

Quality

A major function of the specialty of Radiology is the provision of information on diagnostic studies that patients have undergone at the request of clinicians to assist in the management of their care. Essential qualities of this service are: a) timeliness and b) accuracy of the information delivered. Several programs have been developed in the department to measure the success of attaining these objectives.

Timeliness
Four programs have been initiated to evaluate the timeliness of the diagnostic report:
1. attending report sign-off time (SOT);
2. turnaround times for diagnostic studies from time of order request entry (TAT);

3. critical information delivery time (CID);
4. spine imaging turn-around time (SIT).
 These will be individually described.

SOT

This program has been in existence for more than 5 years, and it has undergone refinement over that time. 'SOT' refers to the time between the issuing of a preliminary report and the attending radiologist sign-off. The attending radiologist is provided, on a quarterly basis, the mean number of hours of their conduct, and the mean of the department as a whole. There has been steady improvement in the attending sign-off over recent years, with the percentage of cases signed off at 0–2 hours increasing from 51.1% in fiscal year (FY) 2010, to 66.1% in FY 2011, and 70.8% in FY 2012.

A number of factors have accounted for this great improvement—noteworthy is the adoption of speech-recognition software—however, a major contributing factor has been that the department has recorded these values and made it available to attending radiologists to guide them to improve their performance to match or improve upon the values of the department as a whole. In many respects, the success of this program has served as the model for subsequent, quantitative, number-based assessments.

TAT

This program was expanded and promulgated approximately 1.5 years ago. The metric that is currently evaluated is the time between order entry for the imaging study and the issuance of a preliminary report. The concept is the time between when a clinician orders a study and first gets report of the findings (on the radiology information system [RIS]). The current goal established is that 80% of studies achieve this within 90 minutes. Based on these data, members of the quality team have been able to present meaningful numbers to the constituent members of the radiology imaging team (including technologists and radiologists) in order to identify problem sites for time delay and guide future improvement. This has been an ongoing success.

At the present time studies that originate from the emergency department (ED) are subjected to this evaluation. The individual modalities of computed tomography (CT), magnetic resonance imaging (MRI), ultrasound (US), and plain films (PF) are individually examined. Of these modalities, currently the most reliable data are generated from CT, reflecting

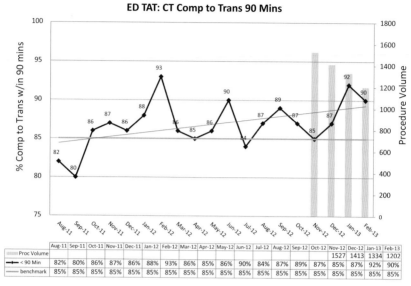

	Aug-11	Sep-11	Oct-11	Nov-11	Dec-11	Jan-12	Feb-12	Mar-12	Apr-12	May-12	Jun-12	Jul-12	Aug-12	Sep-12	Oct-12	Nov-12	Dec-12	Jan-13	Feb-13
Proc Volume																1527	1413	1334	1202
< 90 Min	82%	80%	86%	87%	86%	88%	93%	86%	85%	86%	90%	84%	87%	89%	87%	85%	87%	92%	90%
benchmark	85%	85%	85%	85%	85%	85%	85%	85%	85%	85%	85%	85%	85%	85%	85%	85%	85%	85%	85%

Figure 8.1 Time of order request entry (TAT) program: Time between clinician's study order and delivery of report of the findings. The current goal established is that 80% of studies achieve this within 90 minutes. (See color plate 8.1.) *Courtesy of Dave Tourville, MHA, Radiology Support Manager, Department of Radiology, University of North Carolina at Chapel Hill, NC, USA.*

the fact that there are large numbers of these performed and the data are thereby more reliable and consistent for statistical evaluation.

The goal of 80% of CT studies meeting our TAT requirement has been met consistently over the last 23 months (Figure 8.1).

Future plans involve more advanced evaluation of the various imaging modalities, including: further subdivision into body region of exams (e.g. CT subdivided into head, spine, extremity, chest, abdomen, and pelvis); more detailed subdivision of time points in the imaging chain; additional evaluation of inpatient and outpatient examinations; and superior display methods for data acquired. Many of these goals will be achievable with the initiation of the new RIS system.

CID

This program has been developed to ensure that disease processes that may be life threatening are directly communicated verbally to members of the study ordering team. Our current goal is that all cases should be informed verbally within 60 minutes of study completion, and verification of this is established by computer tracking by the Hospital Radiology Safety Officer, who tracks the codes for critical findings and examines the report

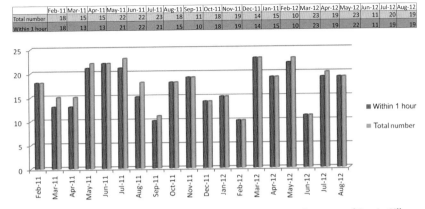

	Feb-11	Mar-11	Apr-11	May-11	Jun-11	Jul-11	Aug-11	Sep-11	Oct-11	Nov-11	Dec-11	Jan-11	Feb-12	Mar-12	Apr-12	May-12	Jun-12	Jul-12	Aug-12
Total number	18	15	15	22	22	23	18	11	18	19	14	15	10	23	19	23	11	20	19
Within 1 hour	18	13	13	21	22	21	15	10	18	19	14	15	10	23	19	22	11	19	19

Figure 8.2 Critical information delivery (CID) time program. Courtesy of Davia Silberman, RT, Department of Radiology, University of North Carolina at Chapel Hill, NC, USA.

for the specific description that the ordering team has been contacted at a described time. In cases in which a verbal description is not acknowledged to have occurred in the report, or where it fell outside the 60 minutes, the safety officer brings them to the attention of the Vice Chair for Quality and Safety, who discusses directly with the interpreting Radiology resident and attending to determine the cause of the delay. The resolution is then reported back to the safety officer.

At the present time the goal of CID has been met with 95% to 100% success rate for at least the last 6 months. Figure 8.2 demonstrates the last 18 months of CID data in tabular and graphic display.

SIT

This is a very new program that has been in effect for approximately 3 months. This study has been initiated by members of the trauma team to meet their accreditation requirements as a recognized trauma center. Radiology has been working in collaboration with this group in order that we deliver to them the data that they need, and also to specifically gear our practice to fulfill their requirements. The current principle metric that is evaluated is the time between order entry for a spine study for a potentially unstable spine and the time that the radiology attending signs off on that study. In discussions with the trauma team, members of the Radiology team were made aware of their requirement. On this basis, modification has been made of attending practice in neuroradiology, where spine studies are prioritized to obtain early sign-off. Additional programs involving the brain are also in development in the Department of Radiology to meet the requirements both of the hospital and of specific specialties to meet their accreditation requirements. We anticipate that radiology departments throughout the USA—in fact throughout the world—will need to act in unison with other departments, who, because of their heavy reliance on radiological findings to make important clinical decisions, will need compliance with Radiology in order to meet their own accreditation needs from various regulatory bodies. We believe it is essential that radiology departments work closely with other departments to achieve their goals, provided of course that they are reasonable, as this further strengthens the importance of Radiology in an institution, and that radiology functions cannot simply be outsourced to the lowest bidder.

Diagnostic accuracy of reports

Three programs have been established to evaluate diagnostic accuracy of reports: 1) morbidity and mortality rounds (M&M); 2) random review of imaging reports that have been previously reported (RIR); and 3) anonymous evaluation of radiologist performance by clinical physicians (AER).

M&M

M&M have been established components of the subspecialty programs of neuroradiology, mammography, and interventional radiology for many years at our centers and worldwide, and have been performed by abdominal imaging for many years as part of their radiology–pathology teaching sessions. Over the previous 2 years biannual M&M for the entire department has been performed with variable success. Currently a department-wide M&M has been formally established under the auspices of the Program Director and Vice Chair of Quality and Safety, where every 2 months M&M is presented, led by differing subsections in Radiology on a rotational basis. In the current era of expanded demands on radiologists' times, in our view it is important to send out reminders, perhaps quarterly email reminders, about various aspects of citizenship in the department of Radiology that senior management considers important. Attendance of faculty at M&M may be one of those functions.

RIR

Currently the department employs a commercially available product to conduct RIR, termed RadPeer, which is a product developed by the American College of Radiology. A number of sections in the department employ

RadPeer. Programs of this type are considered of value to ensure continued accreditation of the center as a center of excellence, which may impact the willingness of insurers to pay for studies performed at a center. The program of RadPeer is overseen by the Departmental Quality Officer under the supervision of the Vice Chair of Quality and Safety. Use of this has been ongoing for more than 3 years, and it has been met with conditional success. There are problems with the product, including that it is cumbersome and is standalone, the interpretations of accuracy of reports are subjective, no direct feedback goes to the individual involved, and it is unclear how problem cases are managed by the American College of Radiology (ACR).

To describe the program and how it is employed in the department: on a specific day of the week the interpreting radiologist reviews the most recent previous case (if one exists) of a study that is being interpreted and assesses their level of agreement of the dictation on the prior case using the following scale: 1) complete agreement, 2) agreement with minor differences, 3) agreement with potentially important disagreement, and 4) predominantly disagreement. Reports that generate a rating of 3) and 4) are transmitted back to the ACR. We imagine that other centers may have similar issues with RadPeer, but others with a greater emphasis on this metric of quality evaluation may have it more seamlessly integrated into their workflow. We can only imagine that our issues are probably in the majority.

The future plan with RIR is to employ a program that can be directly incorporated into the RIS to ease use, and in which the cases evaluated can be more easily tracked and evaluated. A program that accomplishes this is peerVue, and the current plan is to incorporate this into our new institutional RIS.

An alternative approach to accomplish RIR is objective determination of radiologist performance using blinded outside reads, which has been pioneered and published by the Vice Chair of Quality and Safety [3].

This approach is time-intensive and has achieved considerable national and international use in the setting of medicolegal cases to determine standard of care [3]. Although this is a useful tool, it is not currently used as a daily assessment tool for general quality in the Department of Radiology. There is, however, no reason that this program should not be implemented on a more regular basis, especially as it provides data that can be considered objective for individuals in the department whose competency has come into question. This subject is also discussed in Chapter 9 (Medicolegal Reform).

AER

Assessment of the quality of service is a concern of considerable interest to virtually all employment endeavors. Borrowing from research into the assessment of teachers in grade school, the Vice Chair of Quality and Safety developed and implemented a to-date novel strategy to assess the performance of attending radiologists: anonymous survey in the perform-ance of radiologists. This survey is developed as a short 4 question survey that is sent out to the customers of Radiology, namely the clinicians that order studies to be performed and interpreted in our department. The survey asks about the following issues: knowledge of the radiologist, accu-racy of the report, timeliness of communication, and collegiality. To attempt to ensure adequate feedback the survey was deliberately designed to take less than 2 minutes (Figure 8.3). Unlike the situation with school-teachers, in which well-informed feedback into performance is challeng-ing, in the case of radiologists the questionnaires are all sent to highly educated professionals, the referring physicians, from whom high-quality responses are anticipated. The numerical grading of these assessments allows for easy display of radiologist performance. The plan is that the radiologist will be provided with their numerical scores and also the scores of the mean of the department, so that they can use this to guide their improvement. The intention is that each attending member should at least have a rating of 5 as a mean, with the expectation that this be elevated

Please complete the following anonymous survey regarding the work performance of the above Radiologist.

Rating scale: 1=Poor; 10=Excellent

1. Does the Radiologist display relevant medical knowledge?	N/A	1	2	3	4	5	6	7	8	9	10
Choose one:	O	O	O	O	O	O	O	O	O	O	O
2. Are diagnostic reports accurate?	N/A	1	2	3	4	5	6	7	8	9	10
Choose one:	O	O	O	O	O	O	O	O	O	O	O
3. Are findings appropriately communicated?	N/A	1	2	3	4	5	6	7	8	9	10
Choose one:	O	O	O	O	O	O	O	O	O	O	O
4. Is the Radiologist professional and collegial with health care workers?	N/A	1	2	3	4	5	6	7	8	9	10
Choose one:		O	O	O	O	O	O	O	O	O	O

Figure 8.3 Anonymous evaluation of radiologist performance: Survey data sheet.

to 7 within the next 2–3 years. It is not clear to what extent poor performance may be used for disciplinary means, but clearly this objective data
does allow for that.

The above summarizes the major quality programs of our Department
of Radiology. Additional smaller projects are ongoing, either as part of the
research interests of individual faculty members or as alternative requirements for Radiology residency. These are beyond the scope of this chapter,
but as they come to mature and result in useful and perhaps important
metrics, these will be included in our global programs.

Safety

The major aspects of safety that are in the direct purview of radiologists
are: 1) safety of the imaging modalities; 2) safety of contrast agents used
in imaging studies; 3) contrast use in patients with renal failure; and 4)
management of acute medical events following contrast administration.
All these subjects are addressed in our safety program and will be described
in brief below.

Safety of imaging modalities

Historically, including to the present time, the major concern of safety in
imaging modalities has been radiation exposure from the use of ionizing
radiation, primarily X-rays, as used in plain radiography and CT, and
gamma rays, as used in nuclear medicine studies. Because of the relatively
high dose of radiation per individual study, and the frequency of its use,
both at our center, and worldwide, the major attention on safety has been
directed at CT. Our approach has been to assign authority to expert radiologists in the department in conjunction with the Hospital Radiology
Physicist to ensure *as low as reasonably achievable* (ALARA) imaging parameters for X-ray delivery have been accomplished. Under their guidance we
continuously refine imaging protocols to ensure delivery of low doses of
radiation per study. This occurrence is memorialized on all of the radiology
reports in the preamble section, describing that this attention to dose has
been done.

One subprogram is worthy of illustration. Approximately 4 years ago
one of our radiologist experts in radiation recommended that all young
girls and young adult females should wear bismuth breast shields when
they undergo CT examination. A chest radiologist, pediatric radiologist,
and radiology physicist studied the literature on this subject and undertook

phantom studies in order to determine whether radiation dose is substantially reduced, while not deteriorating image quality. Their findings revealed that there was no negative impact on image quality while radiation dose was decreased, so since then all female children and all young adult females wear a bismuth breast shield when they undergo chest CT imaging.

Attention to appropriate radiation delivery is also maintained for plain radiology, and much of this work is under the supervision of the Hospital Safety Officer.

Nuclear medicine, positron emission tomography (PET) and PET–CT safety are under the oversight of the Head of Nuclear Medicine in conjunction with a medical physicist, which is customary nationwide.

MRI safety is overseen by the Radiology Director of MRI in conjunction with the Technical MR Supervisor and a radiology physicist. There are multiple issues that attention is directed toward, predominantly related to the powerful magnet and electromagnetic and radiofrequency energy utilized.

Safety with US is overseen by the Radiology Director of Ultrasound with the Technical Ultrasound Supervisor. The lowest concern with safety is observed with US compared with all other imaging modalities.

Contrast agents

In December 2006, our center was among the first radiology departments to adopt a wide-ranging safety policy for the use of gadolinium-based contrast agents (GBCAs). This adoption followed closely reports in the scientific literature that described GBCAs as the likely causative agent for the development of nephrogenic systemic fibrosis (NSF), a crippling and deadly disease experienced by some patients with advanced renal failure who underwent GBCA-enhanced imaging. Modified versions of this policy were shortly adopted worldwide.

The policy has continued to undergo modifications and refinements at our center, the majority scientifically studied and then subsequently published [4–6]. We established ourselves as a world leader in safety with the use of GBCAs and maintain that position today. The success of this program has depended upon close working relations with Nephrology, Dermatology, and Pathology, and with other experts on this subject worldwide. Figure 8.4 and Box 8.1 illustrate our current policy.

Currently we have initiated scientific methodology to evaluate contrast agents when they are being evaluated to be added to our institutional formulary. This was initially trialed with a recently (at the time)

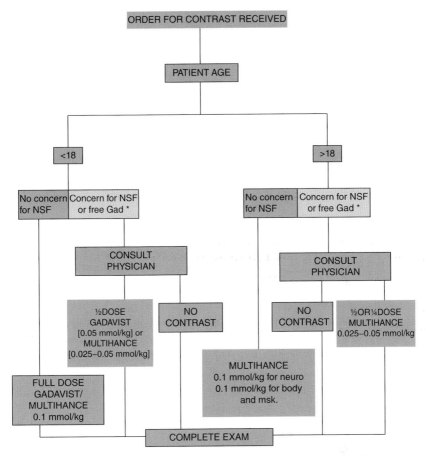

Figure 8.4 Magnetic resonance imaging (MRI) contrast flow chart at the University of North Carolina at Chapel Hill, NC, USA. body = chest, abdomen and pelvic cases; Gad = gadolinium; msk = musculoskeletal cases; neuro = neuroradiology cases; NSF = nephrogenic systemic fibrosis.

FDA-approved macrocyclic (the most stable configuration) GBCA Gadavist. Up until that time, both at our center and worldwide, when new contrast agents have been tested for inclusion in radiology practice at a center, generally the sales person would give anywhere from 10 doses to a month's supply of the agent, and the technologists would use it and report how the experience had been. That strategy is fraught with a host of biases and errors, beyond the scope of this chapter, but among the most important of which are termed the Weber effect and the Lalli

Box 8.1 University of North Carolina Gadolinium Policy

No Omniscan is administered to any patient.

Half dose (0.05 mmol/kg) MultiHance® is to be used on all adult body and MSK subjects. Full dose (0.1 mmol/kg) is to be used on most adult neuro applications, at the discretion of the neuroradiologist overseeing the study. In select liver studies 0.025 mmol/kg Eovist® is to be used, at the discretion of the body radiologist overseeing the study. Pediatric studies are to be performed with full dose (0.1 mmol/kg) Magnevist®. (Updated May 26, 2010).

All patients suspected of having renal compromise, as ascertained by technologist-administered questionnaire, will receive 1/4 dose (0.025 mmol/kg) MultiHance® or no IV contrast, at the discretion of the supervising radiologist. MR technologists have been informed to evaluate patient history on CIS for evidence of renal compromise including sCr, eGFR and other measures.

All third trimester pregnant patients in whom gadolinium is deemed necessary will undergo 1/2 dose MultiHance®.

Gadolinium will be avoided in first and second trimester pregnancies.

No double dose gadolinium studies will be performed, replaced by single dose MultiHance®.

No gadolinium will be used as a substitute for iodine contrast in CT, on angiography, or other X-ray procedures.

Repeat gadolinium-enhanced MR studies should be avoided within 48 hours. If a repeat study is necessary within 48 hours, more detailed evaluation of renal function will be necessary. If renal function is moderately compromised repeat gadolinium studies will not be performed, and either noncontrast study will be performed or a delay beyond 48 hours will be necessary.

Patients with greater than 10-year history of poorly controlled hypertension, greater than 10-year history of insulin-dependent diabetes, and patients older than 70 years of age who are treated for hypertension or diabetes will undergo 1/2 dose MultiHance®.

Patients who are already on hemodialysis should undergo hemodialysis as soon as reasonably feasible following MRI with MultiHance®. A second hemodialysis at 24 hours is suggested but not mandatory. No patient should receive hemodialysis that is not already on hemodialysis, if the indication for dialysis is the MRI study alone.

Modifications of this policy may be implemented on a case-by-case basis when a risk–benefit analysis has been made and the administration of contrast is deemed medically necessary by the attending radiologist. Such determination will be noted in the patient's record.

All chest, abdomen, and pelvis MRIs are to receive 1/2 dose MultiHance® administration. Select 1/2 dose MultiHance® will be used in other body regions.

Patients who experience a moderate adverse event to MultiHance® should receive Magnevist® on follow-up MRI—with the exception of patients at risk for the development of NSF. A moderate event would include: severe hives, respiratory symptomatology, throat swelling, and emesis. Occasionally hives does not constitute a moderate reaction. A severe reaction would constitute consideration of no gadolinium administration on follow-up studies. See the full intravenous contrast policy for description of adverse events. Record should be made of the adverse event, and it should be brought to the attention of the radiology service responsible for the examination so they can include that on their dictation.

effect. The Weber effect describes the situation in which when a new contrast agent is introduced into the department many more adverse events are observed for at least 6 months; the Lalli effect describes the influence of anxious technologists to induce adverse events in patients receiving a novel agent. The innovation introduced at our center was to randomly use either the new or the existing agent on patients and to blind the imaging technologist, the patient, and the interpreting radiologist on which the agent was used. To employ this strategy it was deemed imperative that all approaches be approved by the Food and Drug Administration (FDA), so no undue risk would be encountered by patients. In this particular study no difference was observed in acute adverse events between the agents (neither resulted in any adverse events in a population of 19–20 patients with each agent). Similarly, both agents were perceived to result in adequate image quality by blinded interpreting radiologists. Details of this study have been published [7]. Earlier experience with subjectivity errors have been observed at our institution for trialing CT contrast agents, so our plan is also to implement this scientific basis of contrast evaluation for CT contrast agents. Our intention is to employ this scientific approach to evaluating introduction of contrast agents into our hospital system, including MRI and CT agents, as we move forward.

Contrast agent use in patients with renal failure

Great care is paid to imaging patients in renal failure with CT or MRI. Experts in our department are charged with paying attention to the literature to determine if new safety aspects are described for iodine-based contrast agents (IBCAs) used in CT. It is based on the fact that approximately 2 years ago one agent, Visipaque, was removed for use in patients with renal failure. Essentially the strategy with IBCAs at the University of North Carolina (UNC) has been to follow the safety guidelines as set out buy the ACR in the annual safety manual on contrast agents. As we are a major research center in the safety of GBCAs the guidelines for our use of these agents is often developed at our center. The combination of our research experience, with the guidelines from the ACR, are used to continue to refine our policies [4]. Box 8.2 shows the evaluation prior to iodine contrast administration used in our institution.

Management of acute adverse events following contrast agent use

Teaching sessions are held at least three times per year in the department by our internal radiologist experts in contrast reactions, supplemented by

Box 8.2 UNC evaluation prior to contrast administration (iodine contrast)

Age: Elderly and pediatric patients are more susceptible for adverse outcome related to contrast injection.

Complete list of medications, including over-the-counter medications and herbal use: Document information on the Medication Reconciliation Form.

Complete list of allergies and reaction symptoms in writing: Patients with previous anaphylactic response to contrast or one or more allergens require radiologist consult. In accordance with JCAHO, 2007. Consult required: Allergy to Contrast: Pre-medication Protocol as directed by the Radiologist/physician designee.

Diabetes: Diabetic patients are higher risk for contrast reaction. (If patient is diabetic on Metformin and has a history of renal dysfunction, hepatic dysfunction, alcohol abuse or severe congestive heart failure, notify the radiologist. Contrast injection is contraindicated. ACR, 2006.

Multiple myeloma: Multiple myeloma may predispose the patient to irreversible renal failure after contrast administration. Consult required. ACR recommends additional hydration before and after contrast injection if contrast is given.

Renal dysfunction: History of renal dysfunction or recent BUN or creatinine level exceeding the laboratory parameters requires consult.

Cardiac status: Significant cardiac disease history increases the risk of adverse reactions to contrast injection. Symptomatic patients (patients with angina, or congestive heart failure with minimal exertion) and patients with problems such as aortic stenosis: Consult required.

Thyroid cancer: If systemic radioactive iodine therapy is part of planned treatment, a pretherapy diagnostic radiographic contrast medium (IV or oral) may be contraindicated. Consult radiologist before injecting contrast. (Consultation with the ordering clinician by the radiologist/independent practitioner is recommended) ACR, 2006.

Pregnancy status: All females of childbearing age should be asked if they could be pregnant. If they are not sure, the ordering physician should be contacted to obtain pregnancy test order. If the pregnancy is confirmed, radiologist/radiology resident consult required.

Lactation status: All females of childbearing age should be asked if they are breastfeeding. Mothers who are breastfeeding should be given the opportunity to make an informed decision as to whether to continue or temporarily interrupt their feedings for 24 hours. The ACR indicates that it is safe for mothers to continue feeding but note that many mothers are apprehensive to do so. Consult required.

Hyperthyroidism: Patients may develop iodine-provoked delayed hyperthyroidism 4–6 weeks after administration of intravascular contrast administration. It is usually self-limited.

The licensed health care provider shall screen the patient for the following risk factors for adverse outcome to contrast injection. Confirmation of patient identification using two identifiers and the presence of the correct order for the correct diagnosis is completed by the licensed health care provider before placing the intravenous device.

a trained technologist expert. All of the Radiology residents have training in basic cardiac life support (BCLS) and advanced cardiac life support (ACLS)—and many of the faculty has as well. All pharmaceutical safety training is performed in accordance with the requirements of the institutional health care system to maintain privileges. Our plan over the upcoming 2 years is to have a more formalized program in safety, with the intention of "walk-throughs" by radiologists in the various regions of the department where contrast reactions may occur, to familiarize them with the entirety of the safety setup. The guidelines used in our department are in accordance with the guidelines on management of adverse events as described in the ACR manual on this subject.

A number of focused safety projects are ongoing in the Department of Radiology, the scope of which are beyond the intention of this document. Projects include the evaluation of interstitial injections of contrast agents at CT imaging, and reduction of radiation dose to patients by various maneuvers in the interventional Radiology suite. The preliminary and ongoing results of both of these studies show that our center performs well, as far as the rate of interstitial injections is on the low side, as reported in the literature, and meaningful reductions in radiation dose are observed in the interventional suite.

Moreover, detailed information of overall incidents that have occurred in the Radiology Department is collected and tabulated monthly, as shown in Figure 8.5. This is essential in order to support future decisions regarding implementation of new programs or corrections in the current programs. Also, this data can bring to attention possible basic problems that may be related to individuals or to the service as a whole, and may also reveal systematic errors. The value of keeping and presenting data as shown is that it is readily understood and trends can be easily recognized, which should prompt action quickly to improve safety.

A major research project has been co-authored by the Vice Chair of Quality and Safety on a study that was performed at a world leading center in the detection of double-stranded DNA (dsDNA) breaks at the University of Erlangen in Germany [8]. The findings of that study showed that the use of an oral antioxidant compilation of over-the-counter substances resulted in meaningful reduction in dsDNA breaks following experimental exposure to radiation. Discussion is in progress regarding administering this oral pill to patients, or to health care workers in the interventional radiology suites, here at our center, prior to patients undergoing ionizing radiation-based imaging studies, or to health care workers on an ongoing daily basis. Details of this study can be found in this publication [8].

	Jan/10	Feb/10	Mar/10	Apr/10	May/10	Jun/10	Jul/10	Aug/10	Sep/10	Jun/12	Jul/12	Aug/12	Sep/12
Falls/injury	0	0	3	5	0	1	1	2	2		2		1
Near miss													
Reaction CT	0	0	2	0	0	0	0	1	0				
Reaction MRI	5	3	6	2	4	6	2	1	3	4	1	1	
Extravasations CT	1	2	3	6	4	2	2	3	4	1		1	1
Extravasations MRI			2				1	1		1	1	1	
Extravasations NM													
Physician error	6	0	2	1	4	1	5	4	1		74	70	1
Technician error	1		2	3	3					1	3	1	1

*Note: July 2012 Supervisors entering ordering errors into PORS

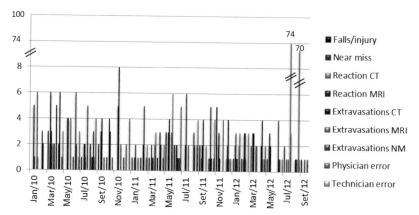

Figure 8.5 Detailed log table and graph of incidents in the Department of Radiology, University of North Carolina at Chapel Hill, NC, USA. (See color plate 8.5.) *Courtesy of Davia Silberman, RT, Department of Radiology, University of North Carolina at Chapel Hill.*

Future directions under consideration include the extent and form in which radiation risk information is provided to patients [9]. The entire effort on safety may also be positively impacted by the use of decision support [10]. Decision-support software is a subject currently under investigation by leadership in the department.

Conclusions

In summary, this chapter describes our experience with quality and safety programs to provide a real-life documentation of the reasonable steps that should be performed to ensure that these goals are being met in any institution. Great efforts are maintained in the Department of Radiology at UNC to both follow the current guidelines of safety as espoused by the leading authority in the USA, the ACR, and to be a leading center worldwide in a number of important safety ventures in

Radiology. The description we have provided above should be considered as a possible model to reproduce elsewhere. More comprehensive description of quality and safety can be found in texts dealing specifically with this subject [11]. We consider it imperative, however, to perform quality and safety assessments that are meaningful, rather than to be involved in complex evaluations that may in fact be rather tangential or avoidant to the essential components of quality and safety.

References

1. Johnson CD, Krecke KN, Miranda R, et al. Quality initiatives: Developing a radiology quality and safety program: A primer. Radiographics 2009; 29:951–959.
2. Abujudeh HH, Kaewlai R, Asfaw BA, et al. Quality initiatives: Key performance indicators for measuring and improving radiology department performance. Radiographics 2010; 30:571–580.
3. Semelka RC, Ryan AF, Yonkers S, et al. Objective determination of standard of care: Use of blind readings by external radiologists. AJR Am J Roentgenol 2010; 195:429–431.
4. Altun E, Martin DR, Wertman R, et al. Nephrogenic systemic fibrosis: Change in incidence following a switch in gadolinium agents and adoption of a gadolinium policy—report from two U.S. universities. Radiology 2009; 253:689–696.
5. de Campos RO, Heredia V, Ramalho M, et al. Quarter-dose (0.025 mmol/kg) gadobenate dimeglumine for abdominal MRI in patients at risk for nephrogenic systemic fibrosis: Preliminary observations. AJR Am J Roentgenol 2011; 196:545–552.
6. Wertman R, Altun E, Martin DR, et al. Risk of nephrogenic systemic fibrosis: Evaluation of gadolinium chelate contrast agents at four American universities. Radiology 2008; 248:799–806.
7. Semelka RC, Hernandes MD, Stallings CG, et al. Objective evaluation of acute adverse events and image quality of gadolinium-based contrast agents (gadobutrol and gadobenate dimeglumine) by blinded evaluation. Pilot study. Magn Reson Imaging 2012; 31:96–101.
8. Kuefner MA, Brand M, Ehrlich J, et al. Effect of antioxidants on X-ray-induced gamma-H2AX foci in human blood lymphocytes: Preliminary observations. Radiology 2012; 264:59–67.
9. Semelka RC, Armao DM, Elias J, Jr, et al. The information imperative: Is it time for an informed consent process explaining the risks of medical radiation? Radiology 2012; 262:15–18.
10. Armao D, Semelka RC, Elias J, Jr. Radiology's ethical responsibility for healthcare reform: Tempering the overutilization of medical imaging and trimming down a heavyweight. J Magn Reson Imaging 2012; 35:512–517.
11. Abujudeh HH, Bruno MA. Quality and Safety in Radiology. New York, NY: Oxford University Press, 2012.

CHAPTER 9

Medicolegal reform

Jorge Elias Jr[1] and Richard C. Semelka[2]

[1] The School of Medicine of Ribeirao Preto, University of Sao Paulo, Brazil
[2] University of North Carolina at Chapel Hill, School of Medicine, Department of Radiology, Chapel Hill, NC, USA

Conservatively, medical litigation contributes at least 10% additional costs to the health care system in the USA. Realistically, the true cost may be higher than 30%, considering defensive medical practice derived from physicians' fear of litigation. The influence and costs of medicolegal litigation go far beyond the actual dollar values attributed to it; concern over litigation pervades all practices of medicine, resulting in tremendous cost overruns in test ordering and drug prescriptions. A vicious cycle of medicolegal action and excessive test ordering (see below) feeds off each other and has established a culture of justifiability. This may be the single most costly component of excess cost in the US system, the least contributory to health benefits of the public, and the least discussed.

Scope of the issue

One important component of health care cost in the USA is the burden of medicolegal costs, detailed in the Joint Economic Committee document "Liability for Medical Malpractice: Issues and Evidence" [1]. These costs include medical malpractice premiums, insurance claims, and medical damages awarded [2]. The perception of many physicians is that the medicolegal aspect of US health care is a contributor to the excessive costs of the health care system [3–5]. A recent study showed that the need for medicolegal reform was emphasized by 12/14 (86%) US radiologists, and represented one of the two commonly cited weaknesses of the US health care system [6]. This perception arguably leads to defensive medical practices costing billions of dollars [7], and exposure of patients to unnecessary

Health Care Reform in Radiology, First Edition. Richard C. Semelka and Jorge Elias Jr.
© 2013 John Wiley & Sons, Inc. Published 2013 by John Wiley & Sons, Inc.

harm, such as unnecessary computed tomography (CT) examinations and the attendant radiation exposure [8]. Concern over litigation also impacts on shortages of physicians. It is well recognized that in many states there is a shortage of obstetrics and gynecology physicians, but within Radiology itself there are shortages in subspecialties that are associated with a high risk of litigation, such as mammography. Although the concerns may exceed the actual risk of litigation, the perception nonetheless affects behavior and clinical decision making [9].

A recent analysis by Price Waterhouse determined that there was approximately $1 trillion in waste in the US health care system, with $200 billion attributable to defensive health care practice [10]. Similarly, Lubell reports, "Medical malpractice costs average about $55.6 billion annually, or 2.4% of annual health care spending" [11]. In reality, due to the pervasive nature of defensive health care practice, the real cost may be considerably larger. In Radiology, it is often observed as physicians ordering increased numbers of studies, especially through the emergency department, than may be warranted [12], and radiologists themselves recommending more additional studies or short-term follow-up studies. All of these practices result in increased cost to the health care system, and increased risk to patients from radiation exposure and downstream unnecessary further investigation, but they also escape detection as evidence of waste and defensive medical practice.

Not generally acknowledged or appreciated by physicians is that before a medicolegal case can move forward, medical experts must be willing to testify that the health care performance in a particular case does not meet the standard of care and therefore that the plaintiff deserves compensation for the injuries sustained. Standard of care is defined in medicolegal cases as the standard of practice for a physician of the same type and training as the defendant in the geographic region where the service was rendered and at the point in time that the service was rendered. The pronouncement whether medical services rendered to the plaintiff met standard of care is established by medical expert witnesses, who are paid by the legal party who has sought the services of that expert, either plaintiff or defense. The opinion therefore may be, and often is, subjective and biased by knowledge of the clinical outcome and by financial compensation.

Radiologists face the challenge of interpreting visual data to make inferences about the pathologic and clinical significance of the perceived findings. The permanence of the data lends itself to objective evaluation by multiple interpreters and comparison of interpretive agreements. This assessment is best accomplished when all interpreters perform under comparable conditions and with the same clinical information.

Error is an unfortunate, unavoidable part of medicine [13]. Malpractice litigation, therefore, has been deemed a necessary way to protect patients from negligence and compensate those who suffer from medical malpractice. It is beyond question that in egregious cases patients must be compensated for injuries, and furthermore that physicians who practice outside the bounds of accepted practice should be held accountable [14].

A recently published study by our research group investigated the current practice of determining standard of care in medicolegal cases by examining whether specific findings deemed critical to standard of care by expert witnesses are identifiable by radiologists blinded to the clinical outcome and litigation [15]. The results show discord between the paid medical expert witnesses and blinded radiologists interpreting the same data in the evaluation of a subtle finding. This difference clearly defined the scope of the problem of using paid experts who are paid by one or other adversarial legal teams. Two critical components of this study were to ensure as little bias as possible in image interpretation and to ensure that secondary readers would actually read the studies. The steps to minimize bias included not identifying any case as a medicolegal case, submission of a number of cases to simulate clinical practice, inclusion of a control case, inclusion of three randomly assigned cases, and inclusion of a matched case of a similar type (major trauma). The methods used to ensure that the studies would be read by the secondary readers were primarily offering $100 compensation and providing a reasonable but short timeline for completion of the reading. We will describe below other strategies to ensure that outside readers do take part in this process.

In a study preceding the above-described study, Ryan et al. [16] addressed the subject of what should be considered a "true" finding, if there is no pathology specimens obtained or surgery performed immediately after the imaging study. We proposed an imaging "gold standard," where if a finding was observed by 80% of the external readers then it should be considered a "true finding." That percentage may vary depending on the number of readers, but clearly in the range of 66 (2/3 readers) to 90% may be acceptable.

We believe a method such as ours can be used for acquisition of expert opinions to determine standard of care independently of plaintiff and defense compensation. A panel of radiologists blinded to the purpose of the litigation and clinical outcome should interpret a small series of cases that include the legal case. The findings in the legal case would serve as a composite or consensus expert opinion, and the results would determine whether the finding is detectable. The importance of the finding would also be determined. The purpose of this method is to answer two main questions: 1) should the litigation proceed? (this question is especially important in cases in which the findings are subtle); and 2) does the finding confirm or suggest the diagnosis? The panel of radiologists would consist of those currently qualified to interpret the same studies as, or to perform the same tasks as, the radiologist in question. Therefore, radiologists who interpret mammograms are held to the same standard regardless of their fellowship training.

In this study, 31 radiologists who had no knowledge of the clinical outcome or litigation did not confirm expert witness interpretation involving subtle findings. This result illustrates an intrinsic flaw in the current medicolegal system that specifically affects radiologists. State medical boards may serve as the source of the independent opinion before the legal process begins, as is the procedure in some states. In that approach, however, the legal purpose is evident, which may change the behavior of the secondary readers. The effect of this condition is uncertain and would be an area of further research. Alternatively, the method used in our study can be expanded as part of a broad quality assurance program. While the legal purpose is served, data from the additional nonlegal cases can provide important feedback on the interpretive performance of an institution or individual. This will be expanded below.

This study was limited by the inability of the authors to describe the details of the medicolegal case in the paper itself, because it was subject to a confidentiality agreement as part of the settlement. Bias against the primary reader was present in the study and perhaps unavoidable in the circumstances of the study design. Standard of care is meant to be determined as a reflection of practice when the medical service was rendered, which in this case was 4 years before the outside readers interpreted the study, and these readers were not instructed to render an opinion of practice of 4 years prior. In addition, the legal determination can vary from state to state.

A major factor that drives litigation, which is absent in other developed nations [6], is that in the USA, health care is not guaranteed to all its citizens. In a non-universal health coverage system, such as that in the USA, if a patient loses health insurance and has continued, often expensive, health care needs, that patient has essentially no option but to litigate against some party in order to get funds to continue to pay for their health care [15]. The obvious parties to litigate against are those with the greatest financial resources, which are often the health care providers and the hospitals involved. Thus, financial need probably represents one of the main drivers of litigious activity, even if the injured party feels that the health care providers are not responsible. We propose that the absence of a comprehensive and universal health care plan in the USA is one of the key factors related to the disproportionate degree of health care litigation. The disconnect between medicolegal practice and quality of health care is best expressed by studies that show that the USA has the greatest affliction of medicolegal action [2, 6, 17–21], while at the same time possessing the best-trained, best-qualified physicians, and the latest health care innovations and hospital systems [22, 23]. Universal health care systems have their own drawbacks, such as long wait times [24], and do not compensate for the tragedy that befalls individuals if they are faced with high health care costs and have no insurance coverage and low-paying employment.

A downside of a system that relies on litigation settlements to compensate for shortcomings in health care coverage is that a relatively small percentage of those injured are able to win a medicolegal case [25]. This phenomenon we have termed "bingo" health care, where one individual may win, by getting their health care costs covered by litigation, but most people lose because they cannot. In addition, a confrontational culture arises from the adversarial nature of medicolegal proceedings, which engenders mistrust in the doctor–patient relationship. A manifestation of this phenomenon may account for the pattern of practice referred to as "defensive medicine"; physicians feel compelled to perform additional tests and procedures, some of which increase costs and/or risk to the patient (e.g. the overutilization of CT) [8, 26–30].

It is well recognized that good communication between doctor and patient greatly assists in staving off medical litigation if a health care misadventure occurs [31], but diagnostic radiologists do not generally have the opportunity to communicate with patients, and therefore represent a nameless, faceless, high bill, when it comes time for a patient to consider whether they should pursue legal action.

An additional, major problem with the nature of medicolegal action is that the findings in these cases are usually confidential, so there is generally little opportunity to learn from the aspects of a case. This is therefore distinct from multidisciplinary conferences or morbidity and mortality conferences held by physicians, where the intent is to improve learning and awareness. We have become aware in medicolegal cases of such topics as soft-tissue Chance fractures, the medial wall of the ascending colon being a common blind spot in colonoscopy, and bowel injuries from seat belt compression in motor vehicle accidents, but as the information is subject to confidentiality it would be with peril that we would divulge to the medical community the important lessons we have learned from other people's (patients' and physicians') tragedies.

Limitations on the patient's side of the current medicolegal system include the fact that plaintiff legal teams are prohibited from providing funds to patients to sustain themselves, when very often, patients who are injured are (newly) poor. Hence the incentive is for them to settle, because otherwise they may not be able to provide financially for themselves and for their families.

Ideal solution

The ideal solutions for medicolegal reform include strategies that increase the ability of justice to be fair and balanced, and to ensure that a patient who is injured receives fair and appropriate compensation to sustain themselves. Articles have often emphasized that a critical component of physician interaction with patients to minimize the likelihood of legal cases, even when health care delivery to the patient has been flawed, is communication and accountability [31–34]. A recent approach advocated that health care systems should employ in dealing with patients and health care mistakes includes three elements: acknowledgment, apology, and compensation [15, 16, 35].

To strive for objectivity, we have proposed approaches such as the use of multiple external blinded readers, who act as agents of the court rather than agents of the adversarial legal parties, to determine the "truth" in a case. As a first level of integrity, the experts should be blinded and interpret a number of cases, in addition to the target case; and as a second level of integrity, they should not be influenced in their thinking by factors that lead to pandering to the adversarial team's desires.

There is also currently a surprising lack of accountability assurance on the part of expert witness opinions. Hence a culture of "saying whatever the legal team wants them to say" exists. This can be readily corrected by holding experts accountable for their opinions. The strategy we would use is a variation of our "imaging truth" formula: if their opinion is not supported by 30% of blinded readers then the opinion is suspect; if their opinion approaches 0% support by blinded readers, then it should initiate mandatory prosecution for perjury. Essentially, if their opinion differs substantially from the norm of the blinded reads, they should be held accountable.

To diminish frivolous claims the plaintiff team should be held financially liable in the event that the judge deems the case completely without merit (as described in the Jackson opinion article below).

Benefits on the patient side, as currently plaintiff lawyers cannot provide financial living support for disabled patients who may be disabled on the basis of the alleged malpractice, the court should intervene on their behalf and determine a subsistence level and allow the plaintiff legal team to provide that for them, as they await trial. This approach may be most appropriate to apply in legal cases of individuals against large companies rather than against physicians, as currently it is common practice that companies drag out settlements for a long time, by which time the patient may expire, and their settlement be therefore less.

If a jury system is used, then the jury must be composed of individuals learned in medicine or medical law, and we would recommend retired physicians and judges. It is difficult enough for physicians in other specialties to understand the nuances of the medical practice of physicians, let alone untrained members of the public.

Financial compensations (tort reform) as proposed by Elmendorf/ Jackson (see below) are also a necessary component of medicolegal reform. A system of universal health care for everyone, or the ability of an individual to be covered by a preexistent health care plan such as Medicaid or Medicare, even if they don't otherwise qualify, may be a reasonable approach, and this determination could be made by the presiding judge.

Workable solution

Tort reform is clearly needed. An appropriate recommendation by Douglas W. Jackson was published in *Orthopedics Today* in 2009 [36]. He referenced a recent letter to Senator Orrin Hatch (R-Utah), by Douglas W. Elmendorf, the director of the Congressional Budget Office (CBO), who offered the following suggestions for tort reform, including:
- a cap of $250,000 on awards for noneconomic damages;
- a cap on awards for punitive damages of $500,000 or two times the award for economic damages, whichever is greater;
- modification of the "collateral source" rule to allow evidence of income from such sources as health and life insurance, workers' compensation, and automobile insurance to be introduced at trials or to require that such income be subtracted from awards decided by juries;

- a statute of limitations—1 year for adults and 3 years for children—from the date of discovery of an injury;
- replacement of joint-and-several liability with a fair-share rule, under which a defendant in a lawsuit would be liable only for the percentage of the final award that was equal to his or her share of responsibility for the injury.

In his letter, Elmendorf referenced the CBO's earlier estimates on the effects of these reforms on annual health care costs in the USA. He wrote: "If a package of proposals such as those described above was enacted, it would reduce total national health care spending by about 0.5% (about $11 billion in 2009).

He also noted that in terms of the federal budget, enactment of these proposals would reduce mandatory spending for Medicare, Medicaid, the Children's Health Insurance Program, and the Federal Employees Health Benefits program by roughly $41 billion over the next 10 years.

Jackson's commentary is that he would add the following to Elmendorf's list:

- a professional review court or panel to comment on the merits of medical liability cases before trial;
- if a frivolous trial is taken to court and loses, all court costs of the defendant should be covered;
- that actual trials be heard by an agreed panel of experts.

Aspects that we would add to the above recommendations are that all medical experts must be presented with data in a blinded fashion to the outcome of the patient and the supposed findings in the study/procedure/operation, etc., and preferably in the setting of having additional cases mixed in with them. This should be performed not only by the defense team of experts but also by the plaintiff's team. At the present time, it appears that a number of defense team attorneys have begun to employ the strategy of using multiple blinded readers reading multiple cases, in which one is the case in question, whereas we are not aware of any plaintiff teams who do this.

We have further developed Dr. Jackson's concept of using an agreed-upon panel of experts hearing a trial case, by recommending that these experts be composed of retired physicians and judges. This is expanded in our section Ideal solutions (see above).

Justice is portrayed as a young female, blindfolded, holding a balance scale in her hand. Currently the legal system falls short of this on many levels, affecting not only physicians and health care systems but also patients themselves. We believe that our recommendations would help put this right.

References

1. Saxton J. Liability for medical malpractice: Issues and evidence. A Joint Economic Committee study. Joint Economic Committee of the United States Congress. N J Med 2003; 100:13–19.

2. Baicker K, Fisher ES, Chandra A. Malpractice liability costs and the practice of medicine in the Medicare program. Health Aff (Millwood) 2007; 26:841–852.

3. Hope PA. Reforming the medical professional liability insurance system. Am J Med 2003; 114:622–624.

4. Mello MM, Studdert DM, Brennan TA. The new medical malpractice crisis. N Engl J Med 2003; 348:2281–2284.

5. Studdert DM, Mello MM, Brennan TA. Medical malpractice. N Engl J Med 2004; 350:283–292.

6. Burke LM, Martin DR, Bader T, et al. Health care reform in the USA: Recommendations from USA and non-USA radiologists. World J Radiol 2012; 4:44–47.

7. Massachusetts Medical Society. Investigation of defensive medicine in Massachusetts 2008. Available online at: www.massmed.org/defensivemedicine. [accessed on March 1, 2013].

8. Brenner DJ, Hall EJ. Computed tomography—an increasing source of radiation exposure. N Engl J Med 2007; 357:2277–2284.

9. Dick JF, 3rd, Gallagher TH, Brenner RJ, et al. Predictors of radiologists' perceived risk of malpractice lawsuits in breast imaging. AJR Am J Roentgenol 2009; 192:327–333.

10. PriceWaterhouseCoopers' Health Research Institute. The price of excess: Identifying waste in healthcare spending 2008. Available online at: http://www.pwc.com/us/en/healthcare/publications/the-price-of-excess.jhtml. [accessed on March 1, 2013].

11. Lubell J. Researchers peg malpractice costs at over $55 billion. ModernHealthcare 2010. Available online at: http://www.modernhealthcare.com/article/20100907/NEWS/309039975. [accessed on March 1, 2013].

12. Fahimi J, Herring A, Harries A, et al. Computed tomography use among children presenting to emergency departments with abdominal pain. Pediatrics 2012; 130:e1069–1075.

13. Kohn LT, Corrigan JM, Donaldson MS. To err is human: Building a safer health system. In: National Academy Press. Committee on Quality of Health Care in America. Washington, DC: Institute of Medicine, 2000.

14. Jena AB, Chandra A, Lakdawalla D, et al. Outcomes of medical malpractice litigation against US physicians. Arch Intern Med 2012; 172:892–894.

15. Semelka RC, Ryan AF, Yonkers S, et al. Objective determination of standard of care: Use of blind readings by external radiologists. AJR Am J Roentgenol 2010; 195:429–431.

16. Ryan AF, Semelka RC, Molina PL, et al. Evaluation of radiologist interpretive performance using blinded reads by multiple external readers. Invest Radiol 2010; 45:211–216.

17. Barringer PJ, Studdert DM, Kachalia AB, et al. Administrative compensation of medical injuries: A hardy perennial blooms again. J Health Polit Policy Law 2008; 33:725–760.

18. De Ville K. Act first and look up the law afterward?: Medical malpractice and the ethics of defensive medicine. Theor Med Bioeth 1998; 19:569–589.

19. Friedenberg RM. Malpractice reform. Radiology 2004; 231:3–6.

20. Mello MM, Brennan TA. The role of medical liability reform in federal health care reform. N Engl J Med 2009; 361:1–3.

21. Kessler DP, Summerton N, Graham JR. Effects of the medical liability system in Australia, the UK, and the USA. Lancet 2006; 368:240–246.

22. Coleman MP, Quaresma M, Berrino F, et al. Cancer survival in five continents: A worldwide population-based study (CONCORD). Lancet Oncol 2008; 9:730–756.

23. Gatta G, Capocaccia R, Coleman MP, et al. Toward a comparison of survival in American and European cancer patients. Cancer 2000; 89:893–900.

24. Brubaker LM, Picano E, Breen DJ, et al. Health care systems of developed non-U.S. nations: Strengths, weaknesses, and recommendations for the United States—observations from internationally recognized imaging specialists. AJR Am J Roentgenol 2011; 196:W30–36.

25. Jena AB, Seabury S, Lakdawalla D, et al. Malpractice risk according to physician specialty. N Engl J Med 2011; 365:629–636.

26. Hatch SO. Invited commentary—it is time to address the costs of defensive medicine: Comment on "physicians' views on defensive medicine: a national survey". Arch Intern Med 2010; 170:1083–1084.

27. Hillman BJ, Goldsmith JC. The uncritical use of high-tech medical imaging. N Engl J Med 2010; 363:4–6.

28. Kassirer JP. Our stubborn quest for diagnostic certainty. A cause of excessive testing. N Engl J Med 1989; 320:1489–1491.

29. Lauer MS. Elements of danger—the case of medical imaging. N Engl J Med 2009; 361:841–843.

30. Smith-Bindman R. Is computed tomography safe? N Engl J Med 2010; 363: 1–4.

31. Berlin L. Will saying "I'm sorry" prevent a malpractice lawsuit? AJR Am J Roentgenol 2006; 187:10–15.

32. Baggett P. I'm sorry: Apologizing for a mistake might prevent a lawsuit. Tex Med 2005; 101:56–59.

33. Hebert PC, Levin AV, Robertson G. Bioethics for clinicians: 23. Disclosure of medical error. CMAJ 2001; 164:509–513.

34. Coleman DJ. The power of the apology: Resolving medical malpractice claims in South Carolina. Journal of Alternative Dispute Resolution 2012. Available online at: http://adrepub.charlestonlaw.edu/wp-content/uploads/2012/06/Coleman-final-edit.pdf. [accessed on March 1, 2013].

35. American Medical Association. An Ethical Force Program™ Consensus Report. Improving Communication—Improving Care 2006; 144. Available online at: http://

www.ama-assn.org/ama1/pub/upload/mm/369/ef_imp_comm.pdf. [accessed on March 1, 2013].

36. Jackson DW. A real call for change: How about medicolegal reform? Orthopedics Today, 2009. Available online at: http://www.healio.com/orthopedics/news/print/ orthopedics-today/%7B8F262E4B-22BB-4B13-99F0-5753BA9019C4%7D/A-real-call-for-change-How-about-medicolegal-reform. [accessed on March 1, 2013].

CHAPTER 10

Pressures on reduced compensation for clinical service

Jorge Elias Jr[1] and Richard C. Semelka[2]

[1] The School of Medicine of Ribeirao Preto, University of Sao Paulo, Brazil

[2] University of North Carolina at Chapel Hill, School of Medicine, Department of Radiology, Chapel Hill, NC, USA

Decreased payments of studies, discounting multiple studies, and related topics are issues that are foremost in the concerns of many radiologists. We emphasize that new models may need to be embraced. Reimbursement based on quality care rather than fee-for-service will be introduced for Radiology, using experience from clinical practice. Value must be attached to procedures such as consultation with physicians on the findings in studies and recommendations for further imaging or patient care. A supplemental billing structure with hourly reimbursement for these consultations should be considered.

Scope of the issue

Although demand for radiologists has declined in recent years, long-term trends point to a gradual (but steady) revival in demand for radiology services [1]. Radiology is an aging specialty, and it can be anticipated that the supply of radiologists will be significantly reduced in the next 5 to 10 years as a result of retirement and attrition [1]. Supply might be further constrained, should medical graduates be dissuaded from selecting the specialty because of reimbursement cuts. Demand, by contrast, will continue to increase as a response to an aging population, as it has been shown that imaging use greatly increases after age 65 [1].

Health Care Reform in Radiology, First Edition. Richard C. Semelka and Jorge Elias Jr.
© 2013 John Wiley & Sons, Inc. Published 2013 by John Wiley & Sons, Inc.

Service contracts between radiologists and hospitals are under stress in today's economic conditions [2]. The pressure on reimbursement and utilization of high-end imaging studies in conjunction with ever-increasing costs seems to point to a worsening scenario in the future [2].

Industry developments and tendencies have created new pressures on existing radiology service contracts. One example of these trends is the shifting of hospital reimbursement from fee-for-service to prospective payments based on diagnoses and inpatient days by Medicare, Medicaid, and managed care, who subsequently have begun to reduce the amounts paid [2]. Another example is the growth of teleradiology, and its impact on the ability of radiology groups to deliver their services, leading to greater competition [2]. Potential advantages and risks for radiologists considering hospital employment, or even other integration models, are extensively discussed in a recent American College of Radiology (ACR) White Paper [3].

Typical concerns for individual radiologists include salary, retirement benefits, time off, clinical specialization, productivity demands, fairness, and accountability [2]. These issues obviously require different strategies in an employment arrangement as opposed to an independent contractor arrangement. But they remain among the top concerns in radiologists' minds [2]. From a different perspective, hospitals want the arrangement to satisfy their concerns about cost control, market share, outpatient imaging center ownership, clinical quality, patient safety, medical staff satisfaction, competition, regulatory compliance, and utilization control [2]. Priorities vary from one hospital to the next, but these concerns usually float to the top of most lists [2]. Moreover, the expectations of patients and referring physicians regarding radiologists' work remains high, they demand the delivery of accurate and safe diagnostic and prognostic information, help to assess treatment efficacy and complications, directly administer therapy, and help to coordinate patient care [4]. As they relate to the health care system, radiologists improve health care outcomes and increase efficiency [4].

Health care reform marched onto the scene in 2010. How the provisions from the Patient Protection and Affordable Care Act (PPACA) will affect health care and radiology remains to be seen [5]. While no one can reliably predict where the future lies, the forces have already been set in motion to push for greater integration and more patient-centered health care. In the foreseeable future, the success of radiologist–hospital arrangements will increasingly depend on tighter—not looser—working relationships, against the current trend [2].

Radiology practices will begin to pay more attention to major changes in quality requirements, payment, and referral base [5]. One example of change in progress, implementation and testing of clinical decision support, is ongoing at many centers, and has the potential to reduce inappropriate imaging without the burdensome time commitment of using radiology benefit management companies [5]. On the one hand, reduction in inappropriate imaging is a laudable concern that radiologists, as patient fiduciaries, should be concerned about, but on the other hand, how much do inappropriate studies contribute to the bottom line, which may affect radiologist decision making on the unintended consequences of decision support? Our approach is to support appropriate utilization even if part of the end result is decreased profit to radiology practices. It is a matter of doing what is most ethical. Despite the interest in alternative patient-care delivery models, partial data survey shows that only a small percentage of physicians in general are currently involved [6]. About 3% participate in Accountable Care Organizations (ACOs), but 5% say they plan to become involved in the coming year. An ACO is a type of payment and delivery model that ties provider reimbursement to quality metrics and reduction in the total cost of care for an assigned patient population. Nonetheless, it is clearly stated by the ACR that one priority for radiologists to thrive must be to perform the most appropriate imaging examination and interpret them as well as possible, in a way that makes a real difference to the people radiologists serve [4]. Moreover, radiologists have much to contribute to the ACOs on many levels, including: selection of appropriate imaging tests, educational role in their communities in discussing what is more appropriate, support primary care providers helping to reduce specialists referrals, and discussion of contractual relationships [7]. Recommendations have been issued by the ACR describing several ways radiologists might participate in an ACO, and among one of the most important is to act as patient advocates to prevent undue restrictions on well-indicated imaging [7].

In Radiology, non-insurance covered or cash-only practices have largely been confined to whole-body imaging. Whole-body computed tomography (CT) imaging has been in existence for about 10 years. Shopping mall whole-body CT scanning famously was part of the trend of these businesses, where for $1000–2000 one could go in and get one's entire body looked at. Many of these centers fell out of favor about 4 years ago, as it became publicized that medical radiation from CT may cause cancer, and that the nonspecific nature of findings on whole-body CT often lead to an expensive and unwarranted avalanche of further studies and medical therapies. Our preferred approach for this concierge-type medical imaging practice has always been whole-body MRI. Whole-body MRI is much preferred over CT, as it is safer (no ionizing radiation) and is much more accurate, so does not result in further unnecessary testing and treatments to the same extent. A number of MRI experts perform some form of whole-body screening on themselves as proof of the value of this approach. Although we advocate the value of whole-body MRI [8, 9], we do believe that this should remain for the present a noninsurance-covered procedure for the great majority of individuals. This may change when genetic testing in the future may reveal individuals at greater risk for a disease, rather than actually having clinically manifest disease, and this cancer-preventive or early-cancer-detection type indication for MRI may be a valuable and cost-effective clinical approach. In the meantime, if one has the money, detecting a malignant disease before it becomes large and inoperable, is not such a bad idea, if the technique is safe (MRI) and one can afford it.

Another modern trend in health care is that patients are becoming more savvy consumers, and will often look up online hospitals and physicians. Expert doctors will often get numerous emails from patients about health care issues. Dr Semelka frequently gets many emails, especially from mothers describing their experience with having CT studies performed on their children, and it not being explained at the time that there are cancer risks associated with CT. In their subsequent readings, they learn about cancer risks, and they consider that the risks of cancer from the CT(s) their children have undergone are high, and they are often devastated by the fact their children now may have a cancer death sentence due to having undergone CT. The great majority of times, correctly, and responsibly, he counsels them that the amount of radiation so far that their child has received is not excessive, and he personally would not be overly concerned if his own children experienced that radiation, and just be vigilant in the future to not let their children undergo unnecessary CT. The emphasis is made that CT in the setting of major trauma may, however, be life-saving, so this is one indication not to avoid CT.

In the past, most doctors did not discuss treatment costs with patients, but times have changed. Overall, doctors now talk about more than clinical treatment with patients. Just over one-third of physicians (38%) regularly discuss the issue with patients. Almost one half of physicians (46%) said they occasionally discuss cost of care issues if patients raise the subject. This may have a future impact on Radiology. The discussion of cost has historically been between radiologists and insurance carriers, but in the future this may be between referring physicians and their patients, if the costs of expensive imaging get shifted more often on to larger numbers of patients. Patients may choose the cheaper study, and may also chose the imaging facility that charges the lower amount for the same study.

Ideal solution

The ideal solution for health care reimbursement probably reflects a more homogeneous and universal payment system for services rendered. Pay performance for quality care is an important aspect of that, though, and centers/radiologists should be rewarded if fewer inappropriate studies are performed. This would involve a calculation, as we have proposed in Chapter 2, where appropriateness of studies are measured, emphasizing that studies in which the vast majority of times a particular indication results in a normal study (for example, head-ache and head CT) should be dramatically curtailed. Radiologists should also be reimbursed for the value added to patient-centered health care delivery. Some kind of hourly consultation fee for discussion of cases that have already been interpreted, for recommendations for further imaging, and for involvement in multidisciplinary conferences. The lack of reimbursement of consultation negatively impacts on the incomes of radiologists at major centers, especially university centers, as more of their time is devoted to these forms of activities, in comparison with radiologists at freestanding imaging centers.

Workable solution

Subcontractual arrangements for reimbursement are indicative of how unworkable financial formulations for reimbursement are in Radiology, such that they are rendered more and more complex. A current turmoil in Radiology is the discussion of discounting second diagnostic tests by 25–50% in patients receiving one diagnostic bill in a one-day period. This will have the greatest impact on settings where two regions are being imaging together by the same modality, such as abdomen and pelvis CT.

Our opinion is that, as in most things in life, the simpler the solution, the more workable it is. The reimbursement schemes for health care have become like the US tax code: byzantine and inscrutable. There should be fixed prices that are charged for various services by providers, and all insurance carriers and payers reimburse that set charge. Ultimately, this may point toward a single payer system. At the present time, a system exists in which a person charges a certain amount, and routinely this is discounted by 50% by most payers, some pay more, some pay less, also somewhat arbitrarily, and all try to avoid payment altogether in a "gotcha" type scheme. In a recent comprehensive article published in Time Magazine ("Bitter Pill: Why Medical Bills Are Killing Us") by Steven Brill, detailed documentation is presented from patients' hospital bills showing how costs can rise up to 400% per item in a treatment plan [10]. Actually, he correctly states that when debating health care policy the correct question is not "Who should pay the bill?" but "Why exactly are the bills so high?" [10].

Another interesting article by Cheryl Proval covering a presentation from Frank Lexa called "Healthcare Reform and the Future of Radiology: Navigating the Change" at the inaugural ACR® Radiology Leadership Institute™ in Evanston, Illinois, on July 14, 2012 describes many worthwhile issues [11]. One is related to challenges that created the need for health care reform [11]: 1) health care inflation; 2) demographics and the aging of the baby boomers, the generation now transitioning from being net payors into the US Treasury to net recipients; 3) multidirectional fiscal pressure; 4) value; 5) social justice, including the need to extend coverage to 30 million uninsured patients; and 6) the need to shift power from specialty care to primary care.

Considering the "value" issue, it is interesting to note that there are differentiated spending levels depending purely on the zip codes [11]. Examples of health care overutilization can be found throughout the country. The now famous/infamous example is that of the Texas town McAllen, which stands as the lowest USA household income, but has the second most expensive USA health care market, spending twice the national average [12, 13]. In fact, patients in McAllen get more diagnostic testing, more hospital treatment, more surgery, and more home care compared to any another town, and, remarkably, hospital administrators apparently have no recognition of that fact [12, 13]. In these cases, despite the higher expenditure there was no companion increase in quality of health care and population well-being.

Thus, the workable solution will necessitate a higher commitment on the parts of radiologists, radiologists' groups and academy societies to adopt or conform to ACOs models by an active participation in all levels of decisions; with a focus on promoting the added value of well integrated Radiology into health care systems.

Conclusions

In summary, we have briefly provided an overview financial issues that relate to Radiology. The problem with continuously trying to make small corrections to a system that is no longer effective in the current market conditions, is that one gets a patchwork quilt which becomes progressively complex, expensive, and unmanageable. We have also raised the concept that radiologists should be reimbursed for the consultation services that they already currently perform gratis, as part of new formulations of financial compensation for physicians in the evolving financial environment of health care, with an emphasis on quality care over quantity care. Moreover, the importance of Radiology to the effective functioning of the entire health care system must be constantly promoted, and the need for these continuing efforts must also form part of the education of new generations of radiologists.

References

1. Regents Health Resources. The radiology staffing market, temporary and permanent. Radiology Business Journal, 2011. Available online at: http://www.imagingbiz.com/articles/rbj/the-radiology-staffing-market-temporary-and-permanent [accessed on March 1, 2013].
2. Boden TW. Hospital employment—can it work for radiologists? Radiology Today 2012; 13:18. Available online at: http://www.radiologytoday.net/archive/rt0312p18.shtml [accessed on March 1, 2013].
3. Medverd JR, Muroff LR, Brant-Zawadzki MN, Lexa FJ, Levin DC. ACR white paper: New practice models–hospital employment of radiologists: a report from the ACR Future Trends Committee. J Am Coll Radiol 2012; 9:782–787.
4. Gunderman RB, Weinreb JC, Van Moore A, Jr., Hillman BJ, Neiman HL, Thrall JH. Radiology practice models: the 2008 ACR Forum. J Am Coll Radiol 2008; 5:960–964.
5. Vasko C. Health-care Reform and Radiology: Introduction. ImagingBiz, 2011. Available online at: http://www.imagingbiz.com/articles/view/health-care-reform-and-radiology-introduction [accessed on March 1, 2013].
6. Kane L. Medscape Physician Compensation Report: 2012 Results. Available online at: http://www.medscape.com/features/slideshow/compensation/2012/public[accessed on March 6, 2013].
7. Breslau J, Lexa FJ. A radiologist's primer on accountable care organizations. J Am Coll Radiol 2011; 8:164–168.
8. Lauenstein TC, Semelka RC. Whole-body magnetic resonance imaging. Top Magn Reson Imaging 2005; 16:15–20.

9. Hernandes MA, Semelka RC, Elias Jr J, et al. Whole body MRI: Comprehensive evaluation on a 48-channel 3T MRI system in less than 40 minutes: Preliminary results. Radiol Bras 2012; 45:319–325.

10. Brill S. Bitter Pill: Why medical bills are killing us. Time 2013; 181:16–24, 26, 28 passim.

11. Proval C. Shapeshifting in the Era of Health-care Reform. Radiology Business Journal 2012:16–17. Available online at: http://www.imagingbiz.com/images/site/pdf/aug_sep_2012.pdf [accessed on March 1, 2013].

12. Gawande A. The cost conundrum: What a Texas town can teach us about health care. The New Yorker's, 2009. Available online at: http://www.newyorker.com/reporting/2009/06/01/090601fa_fact_gawande [accessed on March 1, 2013].

13. Kauffman-Pickelle C. Radiology and the culture of money. ImagingBiz, 2009. Available online at: http://www.imagingbiz.com/articles/imagingbiz/radiology-and-the-culture-of-money [accessed on March 6, 2013].

CHAPTER 11

National health care systems

Jorge Elias Jr,[1] Lauren M. B. Burke,[2] and Richard C. Semelka[2]

[1] The School of Medicine of Ribeirao Preto, University of Sao Paulo, Brazil
[2] University of North Carolina at Chapel Hill, School of Medicine, Department of Radiology, Chapel Hill, NC, USA

Financial coverage is a major issue in health care. It has generally been a political and financial decision that each nation has made on its own. Nonetheless, the USA stands out as the only developed nation that does not have some form of comprehensive health care insurance for the entirety of its population. Successful efforts should not be on the pure basis of saving money, but on the basis of the overall wellness of the population and the maintenance of current health care practices and technology. It is our opinion that a national health care system works most effectively if well-informed individuals who are not part of a political cycle of elections make decisions. In this chapter, discussion will be made of structured performance incentives and accountability as important factors.

Scope of the issue

In 2000, the World Health Organization (WHO) ranked the health care systems of 191 nations. The USA was a dismal 37th [1]. When the Commonwealth Fund compared the USA with other advanced nations in 2007, the USA ranked last or next-to-last compared with five other nations: Australia, Canada, Germany, New Zealand, and the UK [2]. With over 46 million Americans uninsured and an additional 25 million Americans without adequate health insurance to cover health care costs if they become sick [3], it is not surprising that the subject of health care reform dominated the news in the USA for much of the late 2000s to the present [4–14].

Health Care Reform in Radiology, First Edition. Richard C. Semelka and Jorge Elias Jr.
© 2013 John Wiley & Sons, Inc. Published 2013 by John Wiley & Sons, Inc.

On March 23, 2010, the US congress passed a health care reform bill, which does not cover 100% of US citizens but represents a major effort to improve the health care system [15]. The bill addresses flaws in the US health care system, such as prohibiting denial of health care insurance for patients with preexisting conditions and extending health care coverage for young adults on their parental insurance programs [16, 17]. However, topics such as access to adequate health care and safety of delivered health care remain unaddressed.

Within the debate over health care, there has been considerable discussion about the inclusion of a universal health care plan. Those opposed to this idea often cite the projected cost of such a plan. The increasing cost of US health care and the recent expansion of services have led some to predict that Medicare may become bankrupt as early as 2017 [10]. In fact, it has been postulated that health care spending must be reduced by 6.2% over the next decade to maintain solvency [18]. One of the major components of rising costs is the increased utilization of advanced imaging procedures, such as computed tomography (CT) and magnetic resonance imaging (MRI), which typically are linked with high reimbursement rates [19–21]. Despite the impact of imaging on the increasing costs of health care, opinion and original research by imaging specialists on this subject has been sparse [21].

The perception of changes needed to US health care was presented in recently published surveys of imaging specialists, radiologists and non-radiologists, from developed nations including the USA [22, 23]. The survey asked respondents to comment on the strengths and weaknesses of their health care system and specific recommendations for US health care reform.

Perceptions from the USA

The US respondents praised the high quality of care, and the high degree of innovation, research, and state-of-the-art technology making the US health care system one of the best health care systems worldwide. Additional strengths of the US system included fast access to care (one advantage that may not be present in a universal health care plan) and patient autonomy, which was noted to potentially increase the cost of health care with educated patients demanding further work-up with expensive examinations.

US respondents noted that this fast and effective access to state-of-the-art health care was dependent on access to adequate health insurance, which was felt to be largely inadequate secondary to the insurance industry setting limitations on who qualifies for health care policies and denying coverage for preexisting conditions.

The current medicolegal environment was also cited as a weakness. Respondents felt that medical liability is unpredictable, often arbitrary, and a strong player in the overutilization of tests, leading to continuously rising health care costs. This opinion is supported by a recent analysis by Price Waterhouse, which determined there was approximately $1 trillion in waste in the US health care system, with $200 billion attributable to defensive health care practice [24]. Lubell also reports that "Medical malpractice costs average about $55.6 billion annually, or 2.4% of annual health care spending" [25].

The lack of medicolegal reform was felt to be due in part to the lack of physician input in health care policy decisions. Potential solutions were discussed, including capping financial penalties and the financial award to attorneys, including physician representation in all medicolegal policy reform, and establishing an alternative to the medicolegal system, such as expert medical panels.

Perceptions from abroad

An overwhelming majority of the non-US respondents stated that the greatest strength of their own health care system was universal health care coverage. More specifically, this opinion was shared by 12/17 (71%) of non-US respondents, with universal coverage typically including inpatient or urgent medical care within public hospitals but not necessarily nonurgent outpatient care or procedures [23]. In countries such as Spain, Austria, the UK, Canada, Germany, Italy, Japan, Denmark, Sweden, The Netherlands, South Korea, and France, the public system permits that patients are able to choose their physician and hospital [23]. In other countries such as Australia, Ireland, and Portugal, patient choice is available only with additional private insurance. Specialists from Australia, Austria, France, Ireland, Italy, Japan, and Spain consider the quality of care within the public sector to be very good. In fact, the Austrian respondent claims that 87% of the population is satisfied with the health care system. Overall, many felt that the quality of care was at least very good and that the general population was satisfied with their health care system [23].

Although offering comprehensive coverage to their entire population, respondents felt their universal health care system was relatively inexpensive and efficient. In fact, the respondent from The Netherlands stated that their health care system costs approximately 6.5% of the individual's income, with a maximum of $2900 per year for a standard package (ranging from $1900 USD per year for the lowest income bracket to $3200 USD per year for the highest income bracket).

Several of the surveyed countries (8/17 [47%]) report the option of purchasing private insurance in addition to publicly provided coverage. The private insurance holds several advantages, such as coverage of non-urgent procedures, the ability to choose the physician and the hospital, and shorter waiting times.

Weaknesses included long wait times, with an average of a 1 week wait for a body MRI and 2 month wait for a knee MRI in Canada, or up to a 3–6 month wait for a hip arthroplasty in Sweden. Respondents also felt that asymmetric access to quality care occasionally exists. For instance, in Italy there is a clear geographic gradient in quality of services and customer satisfaction, with less affluent southern regions having substantially lower quality health services than northern and central regions of Italy.

Recognized both as a strength and weakness, government control over health care has prompted several countries to require that physicians follow evidence-based medicine guidelines, which was felt to provide an environment for practicing more efficient medicine. In Ireland, the impact of governmental control has fostered the development of central-ized cancer treatment at "centers of excellence," which have improved cancer outcomes. The UK also has centralized cancer treatment, with the 62-day time to treatment rule; patients with cancer are seen within 31 days and treated within 62 days. However, tight government control was felt to give physicians less autonomy, resulting in constraints on the use of technology such as MRI and positron emission tomography (PET)/CT. In addition, the centralized control was felt to potentially lead to a lack of integration between community associations and political organizations.

Despite universal care, patients in several of the surveyed countries continue to have significant out-of-pocket expenses. Countries such as Belgium make up for increasing health care costs with higher payroll fees; approximately 13% of the resident's salary is withheld while employers contribute an additional 25–30% of the resident's salary to fund the health care system. France's health care system is funded by a 20% tax on gross salary; and in Portugal, out-of-pocket expenses are around 23% of total health expenses.

The ability to purchase additional insurance in the private sector has resulted in a shift of the "bread-and-butter cases" to the private sector and the more complex cases to the public sector. Additionally, in Germany, the private health care systems preferentially insure young healthy patients, leaving the elderly only with public insurance.

Non-US respondents felt the best way to improve access to health care for the economically disadvantaged was with a publicly funded universal health care system. Warnings were given to not give up physician independence and to enforce adequate, fair physician reimbursement. Given that the USA has a higher contribution to health care from its gross domestic product (GDP) [26] than the majority of countries with universal health care, warnings were given to strongly consider cost containment strategies.

The increasing costs of the health care industry have left the sickest and most vulnerable Americans at risk. At least 22,000 people died in the USA in 2006 because they lacked health insurance and had limited access to medical care [9]; the number of deaths related to lack of coverage increases by about 1000 per year [27]. With the rising numbers of uninsured people and rapidly increasing health care costs, the subject of our current health care system has recently taken on much greater importance and the topic of reform has taken on much greater urgency.

The debate within the USA has raised the question of whether a universal health care system is capable of providing state-of-the-art health care while at the same time not bankrupting the country. Interestingly, those non-US respondents felt that their nation's universal health care system provided high-quality health care in a very efficient, uniform manner (noting that there are still some geographic imbalances in the quality of care).

The economics of a universal health care system is a legitimate concern, as universal health care is expensive and the USA already spends more of its GDP on health care than all other countries [26]. While, this supports the notion that universal coverage does not necessarily mean higher costs, cost control becomes an even more important issue. Some believe that if all health care is "free," it may lead to frivolous abuse and overuse of services, which would be financially unsustainable for the nation. This may be controlled, in part, with the use of co-payments, which will help put some of the financial responsibility back on the patient, and cause some reflection before seeking health care.

An additional and important method to cut costs is medicolegal reform. Studies show that the USA has the greatest affliction of medicolegal action [28–34], while at the same time possessing the best-trained, best-qualified physicians, and the latest health care innovations and hospital systems [35, 36]. It is our opinion that meaningful cost reductions can only occur if physicians do not work under the constant threat of litigation. This would decrease "defensive medicine," when physicians feel compelled to perform additional tests and procedures, some of which increase cost and/ or risk to the patient (for example, the overutilization of CT) [37–41].

There is a complex interplay between several factors that may account for the difference in perception between US and non-US radiologists in the need for medicolegal reform in their respective countries, including cultural differences among physicians, the public, physician–patient inter-action, and differences in legal systems. However, it is notable that while the great majority (86%) of US radiologists considered medicolegal reform an important goal, none of the non-US radiologists thought medicolegal issues were important limitations in their own national health care systems. In a recent survey of 1231 physicians, 91% of the responders stated that they believed physicians in the USA order excess tests for medicolegal reasons and not for patient care [42]. This raises the question of how the US system evolved so differently from other developed nations that medi-colegal concerns should be perceived by radiologists to be an enormous impediment in the USA but not of any special concern in other developed countries.

Ideal solution

On CNN Fareed Zacharia reported that Taiwan, in its effort to devise an optimal health care system, evaluated the systems of developed nations and decided upon the Canadian system as the ideal system to emulate in their nation. There is a certain attractiveness to using the Canadian system as a model in the USA; they are our next-door neighbors with whom we have extremely close ties in most aspects of our nations' existences, and they are a very comparable nation with a comparable diverse and similar immigrant population.

There are, however, some problems fraught in a simple translation of the Canadian system to the US system. Although the Canadian system views itself as a government-mediated single payer system, in actuality it is a mixed government-system private-payer system, and differs from other nations which offer a mixed system (such as Australia, the UK, Austria, and Germany) in that the private-payer system is not internal to the country but is actually the US health care system. Many Canadians seek their health care in the USA if they want faster or theoretically better care, especially for challenging diseases. So to emulate the Canadian system, one would actually also have to offer a private practice system with faster access and more technology-driven care as well. Also a major problem with the Canadian system, and virtually all other systems that have government-payer as a prominent component (e.g. Germany), is that the government can arbitrarily determine health care policy for political (often financial) reasons and not optimization of health care system reasons. For example, in Canada it is not uncommon that new services and/or equipment are introduced by the party in power immediately before an election in order to curry favor with the electorate.

Our solution to the health care insurance system in the USA is to emulate systems that combine government and private practice. In our analysis, the Australian system may be the best fit for the US population. Australia, like the USA, is largely an immigrant nation and is based upon the English legal system. A critical aspect is that we recommend that health care policies be a bureaucratic and not a political driven program. The decision-making body on equipment and services should be composed of bureaucrats representing expert-physicians, health care policy experts, and legal experts. These individuals would then be the best positioned and informed for such challenging matters, such as to determine end-of-life type health care financial decision making, or costly care (such as chemotherapy), while at the same time to ensure provision of services to individuals who with relatively low cost interventions could improve dramatically the quality of their lives. One report in the *New England Journal of Medicine* described how individuals who put off health care while waiting for Medicare coverage resulted in a higher total health care expenditure than if they sought care at the time of symptom onset [43]. The conclusion of this study suggests that the costs of expanding health insurance coverage for uninsured adults before they reach the age of 65 years may be partially offset by subsequent reductions in health care use and spending for these adults after the age of 65, particularly if they have cardiovascular disease or diabetes before the age of 65 years [43].

The ideal solution, in short, is an Australian analog health care system in which there is public and private insurance health care coverage, in which governmental decision making on services and equipment is determined by a body of experts outside the political system.

Workable solution

The history of the USA is marked with the concept of individualism and the iconoclastic commonsense hardworking attitude to achieving success. However, it is equally important to keep abreast with change, and to modify practices in accord with following best practices. In health care this requires the ability to carefully evaluate the effects of current medical care and be prepared to modify them abruptly, if what is accepted as good care is shown to be faulty through careful study and observation. In our, and many other expert opinions, the global US health care system is failing and will continue to decline. This decline is propagated by people's general reluctance toward change. However, we have reached a critical point in our health care where Americans need to modify this thinking of iconoclastic exceptionalism by nationality and instead come to understand that by carefully analyzing what is going on in the rest of the world we can learn important insights into what we should be doing ourselves.

The current health care structure that President Obama has favored, in the now-termed "Obamacare," intends to use a private insurer-based general health care system for the nation. Other developed nations that have a similar system are the Netherlands and Switzerland. As a number of weaknesses have been reported in the Dutch system [44, 45], the best working model may be that of the Swiss. Therefore, the US policy makers would be well advised to study in detail the workings, strengths, and weaknesses of other national health care systems such as the Swiss system, before the comprehensive implementation of "Obamacare."

Conclusions

There is no substitute for gaining knowledge by carefully analyzing systems of health care from around the world. If we learn anything from Aethelred the Redeless, it is the importance of seeking good counsel when embarking on critical ventures, and the hazards of not doing so. "Obamacare" is determining to use a private-insurance based national health care type system. The best comparator is the Swiss health care system, and experts from the USA should be charged with studying it. Our preference is to use a universal health care system similar to the Australian system, with the critical emphasis of a bureaucratic body, composed of medical, health policy, and legal experts to determine affordable and quality care for all its citizens.

References

1. World Health Organization. The world health report 2000: Health systems—improving performance. Geneva, Switzerland: World Health Organization, 2000.

2. Davis K, Schoen C, Schoenbaum SC, et al. Mirror, mirror on the wall: An international update on the comparative performance of American health care. The Commonwealth Fund 2007. Available online at: www.commonwealthfund.org/Content/Publications/Fund-Reports/2007/May/Mirror–Mirror-on-the-Wall-An-International-Update-on-the-Comparative-Performance-of-American-Healt.aspx. [accessed March 1, 2013].

3. DeNavas-Walt D, Proctor BD, Smith JC. Income, poverty, and health insurance coverage in the United States 2008. Available online at: www.census.gov/prod/2009pubs/p60-236.pdf. [accessed March 1, 2013].

4. Gawande AA, Fisher ES, Gruber J, et al. The cost of health care—highlights from a discussion about economics and reform. N Engl J Med 2009; 361:1421–1423.

5. Grassley C. Health care reform—a Republican view. N Engl J Med 2009; 361:2397–2399.

6. Rittenhouse DR, Shortell SM, Fisher ES. Primary care and accountable care—two essential elements of delivery-system reform. N Engl J Med 2009; 361:2301–2303.

7. Antiel RM, Curlin FA, James KM, et al. Physicians' beliefs and U.S. health care reform—a national survey. N Engl J Med 2009; 361:e23.

8. Gruber J. Getting the facts straight on health care reform. N Engl J Med 2009; 361:2497–2499.

9. Redlener I, Grant R. America's safety net and health care reform—what lies ahead? N Engl J Med 2009; 361:2201–2204.

10. Baucus M. Doctors, patients, and the need for health care reform. N Engl J Med 2009; 361:1817–1819.

11. Hussey PS, Eibner C, Ridgely MS, et al. Controlling U.S. health care spending—separating promising from unpromising approaches. N Engl J Med 2009; 361:2109–2111.

12. Rosenbaum S. Medicaid and national health care reform. N Engl J Med 2009; 361:2009–2012.

13. Sawicki PT. Communal responsibility for health care—the example of benefit assessment in Germany. N Engl J Med 2009; 361:e42.

14. Weissman JS, Bigby J. Massachusetts health care reform—near-universal coverage at what cost? N Engl J Med 2009; 361:2012–2015.

15. Sommers BD, Swartz K, Epstein A. Policy makers should prepare for major uncertainties in Medicaid enrollment, costs, and needs for physicians under health reform. Health Aff (Millwood) 2011; 30:2186–2193.

16. Collins SR, Nicholson JL. Realizing health reform's potential: Young adults and the Affordable Care Act of 2010. Commonwealth Fund 2010; 101:1–20.

17. Hall J, Moore J. Realizing health reform's potential: Pre-Existing Condition Insurance Plans created by the Affordable Care Act of 2010. Commonwealth Fund 2010; 100:1–20.

18. Sisko A, Truffer C, Smith S, et al. Health spending projections through 2018: Recession effects add uncertainty to the outlook. Health Aff (Millwood) 2009; 28: w346–357.

19. Kowalczyk L. Pricey imaging pushes up health costs. Boston Globe, March 11, 2010. Available online at http://www.boston.com/news/health/articles/2010/03/11/pricey_imaging_pushes_up_health_costs/. [accessed on March 6, 2013].

20. Mitchell JM. Utilization trends for advanced imaging procedures: Evidence from individuals with private insurance coverage in California. Med Care 2008; 46: 460–466.

21. Smith-Bindman R, Miglioretti DL, Larson EB. Rising use of diagnostic medical imaging in a large integrated health system. Health Aff (Millwood) 2008; 27: 1491–1502.

22. Burke LM, Martin DR, Bader T, et al. Health care reform in the USA: Recommendations from USA and non-USA radiologists. World J Radiol 2012; 4:44–47.

23. Brubaker LM, Picano E, Breen DJ, et al. Health care systems of developed non-U.S. nations: Strengths, weaknesses, and recommendations for the United States— observations from internationally recognized imaging specialists. AJR Am J Roentgenol 2011; 196:W30–36.

24. PricewaterhouseCoopers' Health Research Institute. The price of excess: Identifying waste in healthcare spending 2008; 22. Available online at: http://www.pwc.com/us/en/healthcare/publications/the-price-of-excess.jhtml. [accessed on March 1 2013].

25. Lubell J. Researchers peg malpractice costs at over $55 billion. ModernHealthcare.com 2010. Available online at: http://www.modernhealthcare.com/article/20100907/NEWS/309039975. [accessed on March 1, 2013].

26. Lexa FJ. Drivers of health reform in the United States: 2012 and beyond. J Am Coll Radiol 2012; 9:689–693.

27. Dorn S. Uninsured and dying because of it: Updating the Institute of Medicine analysis on the impact of uninsurance on mortality. Washington, DC: Urban Institute 2008. Available online at: http://www.urban.org/UploadedPDF/411588_uninsured_dying.pdf [accessed March 6, 2013].

28. Baicker K, Fisher ES, Chandra A. Malpractice liability costs and the practice of medicine in the Medicare program. Health Aff (Millwood) 2007; 26:841–852.

29. Barringer PJ, Studdert DM, Kachalia AB, et al. Administrative compensation of medical injuries: A hardy perennial blooms again. J Health Polit Policy Law 2008; 33:725–760.

30. De Ville K. Act first and look up the law afterward?: Medical malpractice and the ethics of defensive medicine. Theor Med Bioeth 1998; 19:569–589.

31. Friedenberg RM. Malpractice reform. Radiology 2004; 231:3–6.

32. Kessler DP, Summerton N, Graham JR. Effects of the medical liability system in Australia, the UK, and the USA. Lancet 2006; 368:240–246.

33. Mello MM, Brennan TA. The role of medical liability reform in federal health care reform. N Engl J Med 2009; 361:1–3.

34. Semelka RC, Ryan AF, Yonkers S, et al. Objective determination of standard of care: Use of blind readings by external radiologists. AJR Am J Roentgenol 2010; 195:429–431.

35. Gatta G, Capocaccia R, Coleman MP, et al. Toward a comparison of survival in American and European cancer patients. Cancer 2000; 89:893–900.

36. Coleman MP, Quaresma M, Berrino F, et al. Cancer survival in five continents: A worldwide population-based study (CONCORD). Lancet Oncol 2008; 9:730–756.

37. Hillman BJ, Goldsmith JC. The uncritical use of high-tech medical imaging. N Engl J Med 2010; 363:4–6.

38. Kassirer JP. Our stubborn quest for diagnostic certainty. A cause of excessive testing. N Engl J Med 1989; 320:1489–1491.
39. Lauer MS. Elements of danger—the case of medical imaging. N Engl J Med 2009; 361:841–843.
40. Smith-Bindman R. Is computed tomography safe? N Engl J Med 2010; 363:1–4.
41. Hatch SO. Invited commentary—it is time to address the costs of defensive medicine: Comment on "Physicians' views on defensive medicine: A national survey". Arch Intern Med 2010; 170:1083–1084.
42. Bishop TF, Federman AD, Keyhani S. Physicians' views on defensive medicine: A national survey. Arch Intern Med 2010; 170:1081–1083.
43. McWilliams JM, Meara E, Zaslavsky AM, et al. Use of health services by previously uninsured Medicare beneficiaries. N Engl J Med 2007; 357:143–153.
44. Knottnerus JA, ten Velden GH. Dutch doctors and their patients—effects of health care reform in the Netherlands. N Engl J Med 2007; 357:2424–2426.
45. Okma KG, Marmor TR, Oberlander J. Managed competition for Medicare? Sobering lessons from The Netherlands. N Engl J Med 2011; 365:287–289.

CHAPTER 12

Research in radiology

Richard C. Semelka,[1] Michael Brand,[2] Michael Uder,[2]
Michael A. Kuefner,[2] John Stonestreet,[3] and Jorge Elias Jr[4]

[1] University of North Carolina at Chapel Hill, School of Medicine, Department of Radiology, Chapel Hill, NC, USA
[2] Department of Radiology, University Hospital of Erlangen, Erlangen, Germany
[3] Hopecare Clinical Solutions, Chapel Hill, NC, USA
[4] The School of Medicine of Ribeirao Preto, University of Sao Paulo, Brazil

In recent years, much of the funded research in imaging has been in technical research into novel data acquisitions and in data reconstructions. With a current focus on patient-centered medicine, comparative effectiveness, and accountable care, we believe that emphasis should be placed by national funding organizations on practical, immediately applicable evaluations of value-added benefit, quality, and safety in imaging. In addition to greater funding support for studies that compare the effectiveness of imaging modalities for patient outcome (often patient management is used as a useful surrogate), we highlight below in two sections two areas of research that may have considerable impact on appropriate imaging restraint and imaging safety, respectively—in the sections on strategies to diminish requests for expensive imaging at end of life, in our example by use of the HopeScan, and on evaluating the potential role of antioxidants to mitigate the harmful effects of medical radiation, using tests to detect double-stranded DNA breaks to validate their potential benefit.

Scope of the issue

Medical imaging research has progressed rapidly in recent decades, mainly as a result of the development of new technologies and new clinical indications [1, 2], from sonography through computed tomography (CT), magnetic resonance imaging (MRI), positron emission tomography (PET)–CT

Health Care Reform in Radiology, First Edition. Richard C. Semelka and Jorge Elias Jr.
© 2013 John Wiley & Sons, Inc. Published 2013 by John Wiley & Sons, Inc.

and currently MR–PET. In fact, virtually all medical specialties currently employ an imaging test in their protocols for clinical guidelines and management. This increase in research has only been made possible with adequate funding. Although toward the end of the 20th century research resources in academic radiology were low [3], there has been an accentuation and steady increase in the budget for research in radiology over the last two decades [4]. This does not mean that research funding is adequate or appropriately assigned in Radiology; rather, as presented in the message from the Academy of Radiology Research 2012 Annual Update: "While the [National Institutes of Health (NIH)] has endured flat budgets since 2003, funding for radiology research has nearly doubled during that same time period. However, even the powerful momentum of imaging research cannot withstand a −7.8% cut to the NIH. In just a few months, the NIH faces an unprecedented −$2.4b cut from the deficit reduction ("sequestration") deal made by Congress last summer. Although the precise impact of this loss of funding is hard to predict, Dr. Collins testified before Congress that the cut would result in 2,300 fewer NIH grants" [4].

In the beginning of the 21st century, medical imaging research has become an even more difficult challenge for academic radiology departments for various reasons; to cite a few: 1) time required to provide clinical service, related to the shortage of radiologists; 2) diminished income for researchers compared with clinical practitioners; 3) "research competition" by pharmaceutical and other medical companies in their interests on success of particular products; and 4) time constraints regarding consolidation of research results into clinical practice versus advent of newly proposed technologies [2, 5–8]. Despite all these reasons, the main problem faced by academic radiology departments is to maintain the will to build a productive and innovative research program; ultimately their success will be measured by the amount of national funding acquired. In 2006, Dr. Thrall observed that only eight departments accounted for 50% of the funding for diagnostic radiology research in the NIH, which is more lopsided than observed for other specialties [2].

Research: basic, clinical, and translational

There are two main categories of research in Radiology: basic and clinical. This distinction is important, as the needs in organization and infrastructure are very different for each one. Thrall defined basic research as "the discovery and preclinical development of new imaging methods and devices and any laboratory-based investigations, including those in humans, aimed primarily at discovering new knowledge versus testing a drug, biology, or device for clinical efficacy" [2]. Basic research is generally experimental and laboratory-based and can be subdivided into: 1) research directed at furthering the state of the art of imaging, and 2) research that employs imaging methods as tools for biomedical and bioscientific discovery [8].

Clinical research is broadly defined as research involving human subjects for the purpose of studying medical care delivery [2, 7], and can be divided into: 1) patient-oriented research (e.g. mechanisms of human diseases, therapeutic interventions, clinical trials); 2) epidemiologic and behavioral studies; and 3) outcomes research and health services research [2, 7].

Radiologists need to identify necessary resources, new researchers need to receive appropriate training, and investigators need to be willing to think differently than they have in the past about the capabilities of imaging in order that Radiology research play a prominent role in the medicine of the future [1].

Evidence-based research

The sequence of clinical research trials bringing basic scientific knowledge and resources into best practice for clinical use is termed translational research [7]. As described by Thrall "the constrained economics of the health care system have resulted in a raising of the bar for the quality and quantity of evidence required to justify expenses associated with any new service, including imaging" [7]. Evidence-based research is probably the most important aspect of research in Radiology in the assessment of clinical use of imaging, and has been the most overlooked. A great deal of the absence of concerted critical evaluation of the value of imaging can be explained by a combination of factors, among the most important of which are the following: 1) the fact that clinical practitioners often order imaging studies based on their own individual anecdotal experience (e.g. preoperative chest X-rays) rather than population-based findings; 2) the market-driven enthusiasm for novel techniques and imaging modalities (the "receiving a Christmas gift" effect); 3) the general lack of training in medicine into critical thinking and cost assessment; and 4) the high cost of comparing expensive imaging modalities with each other in an environment where this work is perceived by the medical community as nonscience. The importance of systematic reevaluation of old and "well-established" evidence on a constant basis must also be emphasized.

To illustrate the contentious nature of evaluating the impact of imaging on health care, no better example can be chosen than on studies reporting on X-ray mammography. The most current major article on the subject of screening mammography and breast cancer, published in the *New England Journal of Medicine*, estimates that there may have been an overdiagnosis of breast cancer in 1.3 million American women over the last 30 years [9]. The authors spared addressing the potential harmful effects of using ionizing radiation to study the breasts in their stark assessment of the impact of mammography. This study will be widely criticized in the Radiology community; nonetheless, it does point out a serious pervasive problem observed not only in Radiology, but in all of health care: the certitude as to whether the current health care management of patients actually benefits them. In our opinion, this calls attention to the need for emphasis by national funding agencies on promoting evidence-based analysis on the value of various components of health care services. We also consider that this controversy supports two of the main themes in this book, namely: 1) in the setting of uncertainty, it is wise to err on the side of using safer rather than less safe modalities; and 2) it is likely better to detect malignant disease earlier, when it is potentially curable, than later, when it is potentially incurable. If sonography, or even MRI, should prove very useful to screen for breast cancer in specific groups of high-risk women, it should be used in preference to X-ray mammography, when appropriate. We have also opined throughout this book that MRI should be used in place of CT for many applications, as MRI is already a well-established modality for the interrogation for most forms of disease in the body.

Grant foundations

Distinct from the financial costs and incentives of development, Food and Drug Administration (FDA) approval, and selling of a new drug, in general modifications or improvements of variants on a specific imaging modality do not carry with them the potential for substantial economic success for equipment manufacturing companies; much innovation takes place in an environment of a potential zero sum game, as the major equipment manufacturers all make the various types of equipment. So the advantages of MRI over CT do not, strictly speaking, benefit these companies, as they make both MR and CT systems, so selling more MR systems may be counterbalanced by selling fewer CT systems tests. Additionally, innovations or advantages of showing MRI superiority over CT may not necessarily uniquely benefit the company that has sponsored that research, such that even the competitors may benefit from these innovations without having sustained the costs of clinical research. This analysis is somewhat oversimplified and does not necessarily take into account the potential profit of unique intra-modality discoveries or unique imaging systems such as MR–PET. However, there is a greater risk inherent in an equipment company developing a very expensive product, such as MR–PET, as there is uncertainty as to the clinical viability of it or whether the cost will be reimbursed. In-depth discussion of these economic forces is beyond the scope of this book; however, it is valuable to draw attention to the various forces and the complexities involved. In that concern, it is up to the academic radiology departments to take active participation in clinical research to test the safety of new methods and establish their efficacy and cost-effectiveness [2, 7]. Nonetheless, in order to achieve that, funding is paramount.

To address the issue of improving the scientific quality of cancer research, Bruce Hillman headed a collective that was formed in the 1990s, resulting in the formation of the American College of Radiology Imaging Network (ACRIN) in 1999, a successful effort focused specifically on imaging research in cancer. In 2006 the protocol summary on the ACRIN website listed 24 clinical trials [7], whereas now there are 47 trials listed [10], reflecting the continued success of this organization. Other important initiatives that have further promoted the quantity and quality of radiology research include the Coalition for Imaging & Bioengineering Research (CIBR) and the Academy of Radiology Research [11]. The following is taken from the CIBR's website (http://www.imagingcoalition.org): "The Academy of Radiology Research played a principal role in advocating for Congress to establish the National Institute of Biomedical Imaging and Bioengineering (NIBIB) at the NIH. In addition to supporting the NIBIB's growth and development, the Academy and CIBR are committed to supporting imaging research across all of the NIH institutes".

The above shows that Radiology continues to evolve and improve from representing a clinical support research endeavor to fully developed stand-alone research programs. We emphasize that much more effort must be directed at evidence-based research in order to evaluate whether what we are doing actually carries with it substantial benefit to patients. Below are two distinctly different avenues of research that we want to call attention to, to describe the breadth of research that Radiology should be looking into moving forward. The first study is based on patient and family psychology and its impact on imaging, and the second on more pure bench-top that has the potential for immediate translation into important patient care.

Postmodern medical imaging for end-of-life care: A case for research
John Stonestreet

Much has been made of the apocalyptic health care crisis facing the USA in the years to come. Politicians on both sides accuse the opposing party's plan of bankrupting Medicare. It is undeniable that the recent explosion in health care costs will shortly be accompanied by a similarly devastating explosion in the aging population as a result of the "baby boomer" generation. At the present time, 30% of Medicare's annual expenses already service 5% of patients who die each year, and 78% of that cost is spent on acute care in the last 30 days of life; as the population continues to age, end-of-life health care cost is a serious and unavoidable threat to the US economy. Although a high percentage of this cost goes to life-prolonging measures such as resuscitation and ventilation, unnecessary radiological tests also account for a substantial portion of end-of-life cost. Perhaps more importantly, late-stage radiology tests may create the pathway to a medicalized experience of death for many families, without any substantial benefit.

Consider the following clinical scenario: a physician visits with Mr. Jones to discuss the plan of care for his wife, Mrs. Jones. After an initial discussion of Mrs. Jones's condition, the conversation goes like this:

Physician: At this stage of advanced illness, there are a variety of different care options that you may wish to consider for Mrs. Jones. One option would be to continue our current trajectory of *xyz*; another option would be to discuss a plan of care less focused on fighting disease and more focused on your wife's comfort and overall well-being at this stage.

Mr. Jones: We haven't given up hope yet. When is the last time she had a CT scan?

Physician: I believe it was about 3 months ago.

Mr. Jones: Don't you think she deserves another CT scan?

Physician: If you are interested in having another CT scan ordered, there are a couple of questions I think are worth considering given her multiple comorbidities, her dementia, and her overall status that we discussed: 1) What is the goal of the new CT scan? and 2) How would a new CT scan help us to make the decisions at hand?

Mr. Jones: A new CT scan could help us to know whether the disease is really spreading as fast as it was before or whether there is some sign that our prayers are being answered. Don't you think she deserves that?

Before exploring this conversation, let us evaluate our understanding of this family's situation with some information from their encounters with other clinicians. Later, on the same day as the conversation recounted above, the patient, Mrs. Jones, is visited by a clinical social worker. Mrs. Jones tells the social worker she likes to keep her hospital room door open, but she seems agitated by the movement in the hall during the visit. At one point during the visit, as clinicians come and go from her hospital room, Mrs. Jones cries out: "What are all these people doing in my home?"

This urgent plea to have a sense of home during the later stages of life calls to mind one of the many paradoxical realities of modern medicine: surveys consistently show that most Americans want to die at home surrounded by love, but statistics consistently show that the majority of Americans die in a hospital or other institution, often surrounded by medical technology that is as invasive as it is expensive [12].

During the social worker visit, the chaplain stops by, and the patient's husband, Mr. Jones, steps out into the hall to speak with him: "The doctors have given up hope, chaplain, but we believe in miracles. Would you say a prayer and ask God to heal her?" Mr. Jones specifies the kind of miracle the man is asking God to provide, stating that he fears Mrs. Jones may be beyond the help of medicine and that he is hoping for a direct intervention from God. The chaplain says a prayer and offers to explore Mr. Jones experience of his wife's illness in greater depth, but this spiritual support remains separate from Mr. Jones's relationship with the doctor. Mr. Jones thanks him for the prayer and sets off to find out who can put in that order for the CT scan. "It sure would be nice to prove that doctor wrong," he thinks to himself.

Five weeks later, Mrs. Jones dies in the hospital intensive care unit.

This is not an uncommon scenario. Fifty percent of the US public believes that God can heal a disease that doctors have given up on [13], and belief in divine intervention predicts distrust of doctor diagnosis [14], while related belief in miracles and use of religious coping mechanisms predicts noncompletion of advance directives and preferences for more aggressive end-of-life care [15–18]. By contrast, when this population reports feeling spiritually supported by the medical team, these outcomes are mitigated, and patients experience a higher quality of life at the end of life [19]. If the patient's husband had felt more spiritually supported in his conversation with the physician, could that encounter have become something other than an argument over the value of a CT scan? And if so, could that "something other" have allowed for a different experience of death for this patient and family?

In light of the chaplain and social worker visits, two things are clear about the patient and family referenced above: first, Mrs. Jones is yearning for a sense of home at this late stage of her life; second, Mr. Jones is not looking to medicine for his miracle; what he really wanted from the doctor may have been an experience of shared hope, a feeling of personal connection, an assurance that he was not alone. In a word, care. Because Mr. Jones did not receive the kind of care he needed from the doctor, he channeled his angst into emotionally charged reactivity against the doctor's objective stance on the CT scan, seeking to prove the doctor wrong, even though his hopes are ultimately more spiritual than medical.

Reflecting on this conversation and the eventual outcome, the CT scan order seems to be both an example of, and a predictor for, the kind of futile end-of-life care cost that is crippling the US health care system. The task for radiology and health reform should not necessarily be to set up a panel of government experts that could have proactively denied Medicare reimbursement for this "unnecessary" CT scan (likely this will be a path we are eventually forced by financial necessity to take, unless more creative solutions can be shown to eliminate waste without eliminating choice). The ethical mandate for radiology in this scenario is the same as the ethical mandate for radiology in other challenging contexts covered in this volume: transparency and humility. An important part of moving health care forward is for every specialty to do its part to transparently identify and eliminate waste. To accomplish this goal, we must all embrace the humility necessary to acknowledge to ourselves, and to our colleagues across the spectrum of care, trade-offs and limitations to the value of our services in certain contexts. If a CT scan may not be the best answer for this patient and family, what does good care look like in this context, and how can the field of Radiology use the medium of health reform to advocate for it?

We concluded above that what Mr. Jones really sought from the physician was, not so much a CT scan, even though that came to dominate the conversation, but, in a word, *care*. Care, however, comes in many forms. In modern medicine, many have grown accustomed to thinking of care in technical, rather than spiritual and emotional, terms. The care that Mr. Jones seemed to be seeking, though, was ultimately spiritual and emotional. He tells the doctor that he hasn't "given up hope yet," and he says to the chaplain that the "doctors have given up hope." Even though he admits to the chaplain that his hope does not rest on the doctors' medical interventions, he still feels abandoned by the doctor's lack of hope. The kind of care he seeks from the doctor, then, could be characterized as "hopecare," an expression of care, by the doctor, for his hopes. Is this a realistic expectation?

While modern medicine long insisted on physician objectivity in interactions with patients and families, Dartmouth palliative care physician, Ira Byock, opines that for patients and families facing life-limiting illness, loving care from a physician may just be "The Best Care Possible" [20]. Could "hopecare" have been the "best care possible" in the conversation detailed above? If so, how does "hopecare" fit in to the medical landscape, and how could it have changed the outcome of this encounter?

Toward a person-centered postmodern medical paradigm

Integrating the objective science of modern medicine with the subjective arts of premodern healing, the 21st century is blazing a trail toward the future of postmodern integrative health care. Byock's field of palliative care has led the charge in swinging the medical pendulum away from an exclusively scientific approach to destroying disease, and back in the direction of whole-person care. The growth of hospice is a sign that health is no longer simply the absence of disease, but ultimately a state of well-being, even, and especially, in the process of dying. In addition to palliative care and hospice, oncologists and other curative-focused clinicians across the spectrum of care are embracing the challenge of developing vital communication skills for enhanced conversations with patients and families. Through clinical training programs such as "Oncotalk" (www.oncotalk.info) at the University of Washington, physicians learn methods for managing their own reactivity as they sensitively navigate the many challenging dynamics of patient/family meetings. Along with the growth of palliative care, hospice, and clinical communication training, new attention has been given to the spiritual dimensions of patient care, and there has been an increased awareness of the value of hospital chaplains [21]. All of this is accompanied by a corresponding rise in the use and mainstreaming of complementary and alternative medicine (CAM); much of CAM is directly or indirectly rooted in premodern healing systems and spiritual modalities, including the mainstreamed medicalization of a secularized adaptation of Buddhist meditation known as "mindfulness-based stress reduction" (MBSR) recently suggested by MRI investigation to affect neurological processes [22].

Hopecare's role in postmodern, person-centered care

Hopecare is not a new subspecialized silo but rather a girding of spiritual and emotional formation and a quiver of practical interventions, specific to the art and science of hope, designed particularly for physicians, but also useful for any clinician who interfaces personally with patients and families facing the possibility of life-limiting illness. One of the most pressing needs for Hopecare is in situations, such as the clinical scenario described above, where spiritual hopes for a miracle from God and/or emotional hopes for broaching difficult relationship-oriented conversations, are complicatedly interwoven with medical decisions. Clinicians are people too; so all clinicians bring their own conscious and unconscious spiritual and emotional realities with them to these clinical encounters. These biases are not hidden from patients and families, whose emotional vulnerabilities create heightened sensitivities that can be unintentionally wounded in ways that unconsciously increase reactivity and ultimately diminish the clarity necessary for difficult health care decisions. Naturally then, care transition conversations between physicians and miracle-hopers can create a quagmire [23].

Just as providers who have *not yet* given up hope on a fight with disease can find it difficult to decelerate advanced care [24], so also, providers who have *already* given up hope on a fight with disease can find it difficult to compassionately engage miracle-hoping patients and families [23, 25]. Difficulty engaging miracle hopes when medical science has run out of answers stems from an intuition against the perceived moral dilemma of fanning the flames of "false" hope, and a desire to redirect "false" hopes—for a miracle cure—to more "realistic" hopes—for a good death [23, 26, 27]. There is a critical difference, however, between compassionately sympathizing with miracle-hope and misleadingly promising an unlikely cure [28]. Hope Theory conceptualizes the paradox that patient-centered "hopecare" at this critical juncture turns on a nuanced engagement of miracle hope that is paradoxically counterintuitive to many clinicians [29–31].

Revisiting the above conversation between the physician and the patient's husband, Mr. Jones, the physician explains Mrs. Jones's condition and suggests the possibility of considering a plan of care focused on comfort rather than cure. The patient's husband responds: "We haven't given up hope yet. When is the last time she had a CT scan?"

We know in hindsight from the conversation with the chaplain that the patient's husband is hoping in God, not medicine, and he feels alienated from the doctor in his hope. What if the doctor had addressed the patient's statement, "We haven't given up hope yet," before jumping into a CT scan discussion? Is it possible that the conversation could have ended quite differently? By entering into Mr. Jones's hopes, the doctor could have perhaps forged an emotional bond and gained the trust necessary to navigate the conversation differently. Entering into Mr. Jones's hopes is a subjective act that goes against the objective reflexes of the modern medical paradigm. Postmodernism has forced us all to acknowledge the limitations of each of our many ways of knowing, sophisticated as they may be. While the scientific method is a powerful tool for identifying and destroying disease, the same process of removing yourself from the subject to establish objectivity for the purpose of control and manipulation does not bode well for sensitive clinical conversations.

Remaining objective in the conversation naturally leads to a discussion of the relative value of a CT scan at this stage of the disease process, as we witnessed in the original dialogue above. If objectivity requires the removal of oneself from the subject, subjectivity requires one to draw near and make oneself vulnerable to the other. One way to think about this approach is to envision it as a complementary form of medical imaging. If a CT scan utilizes a modern technology called "invisible light" to capture an image that helps to name a condition and recommend a treatment, could a "HopeScan," like a CT scan, use a postmodern medical modality to shed its own form of "invisible light" on the subject? Could both the technological optics of invisible light and the emotional optics of invisible light be useful for imaging different layers of reality, invisible to the naked eye?

Rather than succumbing to the objective reflex to skip over Mr. Jones's emotional self-disclosure that he hasn't yet given up hope for his wife and rush to a logical evaluation of the relative benefits of a CT scan, what if the physician attempted a subjective dive into the unchartered waters of Mr. Jones's hopes? Here is another path the conversation may have taken:

Physician: I'd be happy to discuss a CT scan with you, Mr. Jones, but first I would love to better understand your hopes for Mrs. Jones on any level, whether physically, spiritually, emotionally, or relationally.

["HopeScan"—Hope Assessment: Physicians can be trained to perform a hope assessment in a way that captures emotional images conducive to creating a safe space necessary for decisional clarity.]

Physician (after HopeScan): After listening to your hopes for Mrs. Jones at this time, Mr. Jones, it sounds like the best care I can offer you right now is to support you in your hope that God may heal your wife's body in a way that I am unable to as a physician.

Mr. Jones: That would really mean the world to me. Would you say a prayer for her, doctor?

Physician: I have a prayer here that has been meaningful to other patients and families. You could take it with you after we pray it together if you like.

["The Hope Prayer"—Spiritual Intervention: One of the intervention resources Hopecare provides is a specific prayer that can be licensed to certified providers for this clinical context. Training is required to ensure cultural sensitivity and proper use. Many physicians do not feel qualified to ad lib a prayer in clinical settings, but feel more comfortable distributing a specific prayer in pamphlet form to each of the family members to read together so that the focus is not on the physician's performance of the prayer.]

Mr. Jones (after "The Hope Prayer"): Thank you so much, doctor. I think the hardest part of thinking about my wife dying is that there are some things I need to say to her, and I don't know how to do it.

Physician: Thank you for trusting me with your struggle, Mr. Jones. I can only imagine how that would feel for you. Would you like to explore this further with the chaplain?

Mr. Jones: Yeah, that would be great.

Five weeks later, Mrs. Jones dies at home in the company of her husband. The clinical outcome was not changed, but the Joneses met this fate more acceptingly, in peace and in respect, and the intensive-care-unit bed that would have provided an isolated and technologized experience of death for Mrs. Jones was instead available for her niece, who needed critical care to recover from a car accident. While a CT scan could have shed one dimension of invisible light on the Jones's situation, the HopeScan shed a different dimension of invisible light, with a postmodern diagnostic power that proved complementary to the modern medical paradigm in this context.

If a hope assessment tool and a spiritual intervention could be considered preferential care to a CT scan and extended hospitalization for this patient, then how can Radiology use this branch of health reform to be a part of the health care solution? Are there clinical contexts, like end-of-life care, in which radiologists should advocate for Medicare to require that an intervention such as a HopeScan be performed before a CT scan can be ordered?

As we embark upon the future of health care reform, it may be wise to remember that it has been said about reformers of all kinds that though they may be "right about what's wrong," they also tend to be "wrong about what's right." To be right, not only about what's wrong, but also about what's right, requires a healthy dose of transparency and humility. Most recipes for reform replace careful deliberation with the reckless zeal that is often required to overcome the inertia standing in the way of progress. There is a subtle but radical difference between rationing care and simply ensuring that care be taken to clarify the decision-making process. Succeeding in this vein may require some clinicians to take up Hopecare.com's challenge to "unlearn objectivity" and "do your Hopework" so that they can simultaneously improve health care quality and efficiency by fulfilling the vow to do no harm to the emotion sensitivities of vulnerable patients and families.

As the great success of the modern medical paradigm ironically threatens to upend the US economy, could previously undervalued premodern healing paradigms paradoxically yield postmodern solutions to some modern medical dilemmas? Perhaps that is what we witnessed in the conversation above. While the CT scan's powerful technology of invisible light is invaluable for the purposes of modern medical imaging, a HopeScan shed an emotional and spiritual dimension of invisible light, demonstrating that postmodern medical imaging proves complementary to the modern medical paradigm for end-of-life care.

John Stonestreet is founder and president of Hopecare, Inc., endorsed by the Antiochian Orthodox Christian Archdiocese of North America for service in the spiritual dimensions of health care. He has a wide range of training and experience in chaplaincy and integrative health coaching. His current research interests include evaluating scientifically the impact of the "HopeScan" assessment, "The Hope Prayer" intervention, and "Hopework" clinical training on decisions to order high cost imaging tests within the last 30 days of life.

DNA double-strand breaks as biological markers for radiation-induced DNA damages in radiology
Michael Brand, Michael Uder, and Michael A. Kuefner

Background
Shortly after the discovery of X-rays, their damaging effect on biological tissues was observed. The determination of radiation exposure in diagnostic and interventional radiology is usually based on physical measurements or mathematical algorithms with standardized dose simulations. However, these dose estimations can assess the X-ray exposure but not the biological interaction of the X-rays within the body of the patients. Nowadays it is well known that the biological radiation damage depends not only on dose but also on other individual factors that cannot be adequately ascertained by established methods for dose measurement. A novel immunofluorescence microscopy approach, that is more sensitive than previous biological methods, allows the determination of distinct DNA double-strand breaks (DSBs) in peripheral blood lymphocytes and thus allows an accurate estimation of the biological radiation dose in diagnostic and interventional radiology procedures.

γ-H2AX-Immunfluorescence microscopy
After the induction of DNA DSBs, the phosphorylation of the histone variant H2AX is one of the earliest cellular responses. This phosphorylated histone (termed γ-H2AX) can be visualized by fluorescence microscopy as distinct fluorescent foci using specific primary and fluorescent secondary antibodies [32, 33]. After X-ray exposure, DSB induction leads to a quick increase of foci and a peak value can be obtained within a few minutes after irradiation. Figure 12.1 (see color plate 12.1) shows an exemplary microscopic image of the stained lymphocyte nuclei before (left panel) and after radiation with a dose of 50 mGy (right panel). Using gradient centrifugation lymphocytes are isolated from blood samples and fixed, and DNA DSBs can be quantified using the γ-H2AX immunofluorescence microscopy technique. Quantification of γ-H2AX foci is performed using a fluorescence microscope equipped with a 63× or 100× magnification objective. The number of radiation-induced DSBs is calculated by subtracting the baseline values obtained before exposure from the values obtained after exposure. It has been demonstrated in prior research studies that these yields of X-ray-induced DSBs correlate linearly with the deposited radiation dose [32]. In comparison to previous biological dosimetry

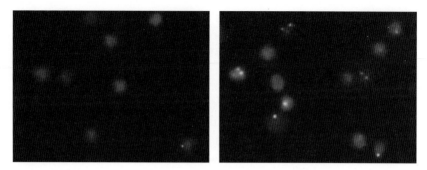

Figure 12.1 Exemplary microscopy images of cell nuclei of lymphocytes after H2AX staining: each tiny green focus represents one DNA DSB. The left panel illustrates non-irradiated lymphocytes; the right panel demonstrates cells after in-vitro irradiation with 50 mGy. For assessment of the number of radiation-induced DSB, pre-exposure levels must be subtracted from post-exposure values. (See color plate 12.1.)

approaches (e.g. pulsed gel electrophoresis or detection of chromosomal damages), this method is much more sensitive and enables detection of biological doses as low as 1 mGy in vitro and in vivo. Therefore, it can be applied in dose ranges as used in diagnostic and interventional radiological procedures. Additionally lymphocytes can also be stained against 53BP1, which is another very sensitive marker for DNA DSBs.

DSBs after CT

In 2005 the first paper was published of studies of DNA DSBs in patients undergoing CT scans of the chest and/or abdomen. A significant increase in DSB level was observed 30 minutes after CT, and then the DSB values dropped rapidly as a result of repairing processes, and after 24 hours the baseline values were nearly reached again. The number of CT-induced DSBs correlated very well with the dose-length product, which is an established exposure parameter in CT [33]. Interestingly, at a comparable dose-length product there was an excessive increase in CT-induced DSBs in one patient compared with the rest of the subjects in the study. In the past, this patient had responded to radiation therapy with very severe side effects, and later a DNA repair defect, which was responsible for the high values of DNA DSBs, was diagnosed (34). This example shows that individual radiation damage depends not only on dose but also on individual factors such as repair capacity. DSB induction after CT and correlation with the radiation dose was also confirmed in another study 2 years later [34].

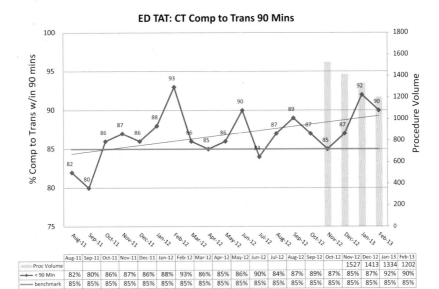

ED TAT: CT Comp to Trans 90 Mins

	Aug-11	Sep-11	Oct-11	Nov-11	Dec-11	Jan-12	Feb-12	Mar-12	Apr-12	May-12	Jun-12	Jul-12	Aug-12	Sep-12	Oct-12	Nov-12	Dec-12	Jan-13	Feb-13
Proc Volume																1527	1413	1334	1202
< 90 Min	82%	80%	86%	87%	86%	88%	93%	86%	85%	86%	90%	84%	87%	89%	87%	85%	87%	92%	90%
benchmark	85%	85%	85%	85%	85%	85%	85%	85%	85%	85%	85%	85%	85%	85%	85%	85%	85%	85%	85%

Color Plate 8.1 Time of order request entry (TAT) program: Time between clinician's study order and delivery of report of the findings. The current goal established is that 80% of studies achieve this within 90 minutes. *Courtesy of Dave Tourville, MHA, Radiology Support Manager, Department of Radiology, University of North Carolina at Chapel Hill, NC, USA.*

Health Care Reform in Radiology, First Edition. Richard C. Semelka and Jorge Elias Jr.
© 2013 John Wiley & Sons, Inc. Published 2013 by John Wiley & Sons, Inc.

	Jan/10	Feb/10	Mar/10	Apr/10	May/10	Jun/10	Jul/10	Aug/10	Sep/10		Jun/12	Jul/12	Aug/12	Sep/12
Falls/injury	0	0	3	5	0	1	1	2	2			2		1
Near miss														
Reaction CT	0	0	2	0	0	0	0	1	0					
Reaction MRI	5	3	6	2	4	6	2	1	3		4	1	1	
Extravasations CT	1	2	3	6	4	2	2	3	4		1		1	1
Extravasations MRI			2				1	1			1		1	1
Extravasations NM														
Physician error	6	0	2	1	4	1	5	4	1			74	70	1
Technician error	1		2	3		3					1	3	1	1

*Note: July 2012 Supervisors entering ordering errors into PORS

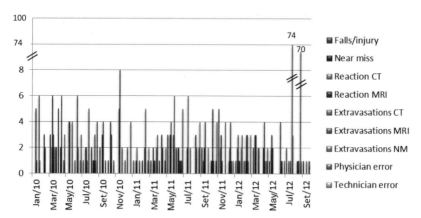

Color Plate 8.5 Detailed log table and graph of incidents in the Department of Radiology, University of North Carolina at Chapel Hill, NC, USA. *Courtesy of Davia Silberman, RT, Department of Radiology, University of North Carolina at Chapel Hill.*

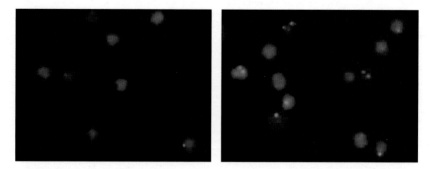

Color Plate 12.1 Exemplary microscopy images of cell nuclei of lymphocytes after H2AX staining: each tiny green focus represents one DNA DSB. The left panel illustrates non-irradiated lymphocytes; the right panel demonstrates cells after in-vitro irradiation with 50 mGy. For assessment of the number of radiation-induced DSB, pre-exposure levels must be subtracted from post-exposure values.

DSBs after cardiac CT

In recent years advances in CT technology have also meant that manu-facturers of CT scanners offer more dose-efficient scanning procedures and analysis protocols. This is particularly important in coronary CT angiogra-phy, because although the scanning range is small, conventional helical scans lead to a relative high dose. ECG-triggered sequential scan modes (so-called "step-and-shoot" technique) or a spiral scan with a very high pitch of more than 3 ("Flash-CT"), allows the mapping of the entire heart in a fraction of a second, and therefore should lead to a dose reduction. Previous studies have shown that these modifications can both reduce the estimated radiation dose and the DNA damage by up to a factor of 10 [35]. In addition, other individual scan parameters also had an impact on DSB induction. For instance, in scans with 100 kV protocols the radiation damage was significantly lower compared with 120 kV. CT-induced DSBs also correlated well with the dose-length product (see Figure 12.2) [36–38].

DSBs and iodine-based contrast medium

Another individual variable is the IV application of iodine-based con-trast medium (ICM), which is necessary in many CT or angiographic

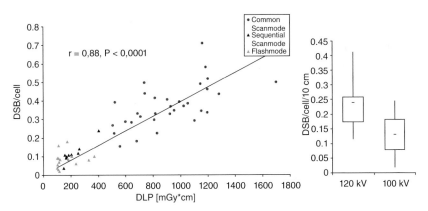

Figure 12.2 DNA DSB after cardiac CT: The left panel demonstrates the correlation between CT-induced DSB and the dose-length product. Values of patients undergoing different scan modes are shown (light grey triangles: High-pitch spiral CT/"Flash-CT"; dark grey triangles: sequential/step-and-shoot CT; blue dots: low-pitch spiral CT). The right panel illustrates the difference in cardiac-CT-induced DSB between patients undergoing 100 and 120 kV scans.

examinations. In-vitro experiments have shown that at the same radiation dose significantly more DNA DSBs were measured in samples containing ICM than in those without ICM or after incubation with various control substances [39]. The addition of ICM immediately after irradiation of the samples had no effect on the number of DSBs, which suggests that the effect can be explained by increased DSB induction and not by disturbed repair. The significant increase of DSBs in combination with ICM is observed after X-ray but not after γ-ray exposure, which is consistent with the notion that ICM increases the radiation dose because of enhanced photoelectric absorption [39]. In the same study, these results were confirmed in vivo in patients who had undergone chest CT; at a comparable dose the radiation damage for contrast-enhanced CT scans was about one-third higher than for noncontrast studies. The cause for the increased induction of DSBs in the presence of ICM can be explained by greater photoelectric absorption in the iodine atoms of the contrast agent and the consequent greater exposure of neighboring lymphocytes [39].

DSBs after angiography

Angiography is a challenging field for dosimetry, because the exposure conditions differ considerably on a case-by-case basis, unlike other radiological procedures, such as CT scans. The radiation is not applied in a single brief period, but fractionated over a longer duration of minutes to hours. In patients undergoing percutaneous transluminal angioplasty (PTA) of lower extremity arteries, a correlation between DSB induction and the dose area product was found—the latter is an established exposure parameter for fluoroscopy and angiography [40]. In another study, following cardiac catheterization in children, there was also an increase in DSBs, but the in-vivo biological dose was not linear in this low dose range [41]; explanation or confirmation of this finding has not as yet been established. Two other studies have shown that the radiation-induced DSBs did not reveal good correlation with the dose area product, but the separate analysis of the various body regions showed good correlation coefficients (e.g. r = 0.71 for pelvis–leg angiography; r = 0.96 for abdominal angiography) [42, 43]. Normalization to the individual dose area product showed significant differences for individual anatomic areas. The damage level of cardiac catheterization was the highest, followed by abdominal intervention, angiography of the pelvis and leg arteries, and the cerebrum. These differences can be explained by the different blood volumes of the various body regions and the associated variable number of exposed lymphocytes [42, 43].

DSBs in PET–CT examinations

In a recent study, DNA DSBs were evaluated in blood lymphocytes of patients undergoing 18F-fluorodeoxyglucose (18F-FDG) PET/CT using γ-H2AX immunofluorescence microscopy. 18F-FDG is trapped within the cytoplasm after uptake by glucose transporters. The radioactive decay of 18F-FDG based on the emission of a positron followed by annihilation with an electron results in γ-radiation. The damaging effect of CT is based on the radiation-induced DSBs. A statistically significant DSB increase was measured in blood lymphocytes both by exposure to the radionuclide and to the X-rays. 18F-FDG-induced DSBs were responsible for about 35% of the total DNA damage induced during the combined PET–CT examination. Peak values were obtained 30 minutes after 18F-FDG injection and 5 minutes after CT. In conclusion, using γ-H2AX immunofluorescence microscopy can be used simultaneously for monitoring of X-ray-induced DNA damage in addition to the determination of the biological impact of radionuclides used in nuclear medicine diagnostic procedures [44].

Estimation of DSBs in tissue

The dependence on exposed blood volume, as described above, shows the limitations of γ-H2AX immunofluorescence microscopy. The method may be limited in assessing radiation exposure of body regions with low blood volumes, as the real DNA damage might be underestimated when DSBs are determined in peripheral blood lymphocytes. This limitation can be overcome in the future by using biological phantom models, where DNA damage can be estimated in distinct tissues. This approach has to be established and evaluated in further studies.

Future of radiation safety: Antioxidant oral agents

DNA damage induction is based on the formation of free radicals. A free radical is an atom or molecule that contains one or more unpaired electrons in an outer orbital. Free radicals are extremely reactive and induce oxidative stress in tissues. Therefore, theoretically an antioxidant should protect the body from free radicals and oxidative stress by donating electrons. Well-recognized antioxidants, such as N-acetylcysteine (NAC), vitamin C, selenium or beta-carotene should reduce DNA damage. The protective effect of antioxidants against radiation damage has been previously postulated. The effect of antioxidant protection against radiation-induced DNA damage had not achieved much scientific investigation until our publication [45, 46]. A commercially available oral formulation, in pill form, of a proprietary composition of antioxidants and glutathione-elevating agents (vitamin C, vitamin E, natural mixed carotenoids [primarily beta-carotene], NAC, alpha-lipoic acid, L-selenomethionine) was studied. In our study published recently in *Radiology*, both in-vitro and in-vivo experiments show that this formulation reduced the number X-ray-induced γ-H2AX as well as 53BP1 foci following an irradiation with a dose of 10 mGy, which is a dose typically used in CT or angiography procedures [47]. In the in-vitro experiments, blood samples were obtained from 25 healthy volunteers with no history of radiation therapy or chemotherapy within the last 6 months, X-ray exposure within the last 3 days, or history of lymphoma or leukemia. Samples were preincubated for 15 and 60 minutes with the antioxidant agent in solution (final concentrations: 33 µg/ml calcium ascorbate, 0.027 IU/ml d-alpha tocopheryl succinate, 1 µg/ml carotenoids, 16.7 µg/ml NAC, 2 µg/ml R-alpha-lipoic acid, 6.7 ng/ml L-selenomethionine) and irradiated with a dose of 10 mGy at room temperature. Cells were cultivated for 5 to 15 minutes at standard conditions (37°C, 5% CO_2, 95% air). In an additional series non-pretreated samples were administered radioprotectants immediately after irradiation, incubated for 5 to 15 minutes and examined again for γ-H2AX foci. For each subject one sample without antioxidants served as control and was also irradiated with 10 mGy. For the determination of the natural DSB baseline levels, non-irradiated samples were used. In order to exclude the chance that the radioprotective agents had a direct effect on DSB levels, non-irradiated samples were incubated with the antioxidants.

For in-vivo/in-vitro experiments, blood samples were obtained before and 15, 30, 60, 120, 180 and 300 minutes after oral ingestion of one dosage of the radioprotective agent (resulting in a total of 500 mg calcium ascorbate, 400 IU d-alpha tocopheryl succinate, 15 mg natural mixed carotenoids, 250 mg NAC, 30 mg alpha-lipoic acid, 100 µg L-selenomethionine). Each sample was irradiated in vitro with a dose of 10 mGy and incubated for 5 minutes after radiation. Non-irradiated samples were used as control.

Lymphocytes were diluted 1:2 with medium, and isolated using gradient centrifugation at 1200*g* for 15 minutes. Isolated lymphocytes were consecutively washed, resuspended in phosphate-buffered saline and spotted onto microscope slides for 10 minutes at room temperature followed by fixation in 100% methanol and permeabilization in 100% acetone. Each sample was washed again, stained overnight using a specific γ-H2AX antibody and Alexa Fluor 488-conjugated goat anti-mouse secondary antibody, respectively. Cells were washed again and mounted with mounting medium containing 4′,6-diamidino-2-phenylindole.

Quantification of γ-H2AX foci was performed in a blinded fashion using a fluorescence microscope equipped with a 63× magnification objective. In each sample, all cells were counted until 40 foci were detected and the ratio of foci was related to the total number of enumerated cells. The numbers of excess foci were calculated by subtraction of corresponding non-irradiated (baseline levels) from irradiated samples, and represent the amount of X-ray-induced DSBs.

In one recent study we showed that the in-vitro test pre-exposure γ-H2AX foci levels in nontreated samples ranged from 0.050 to 0.097/cell; in non-irradiated, pretreated samples, foci levels ranged from 0.076 to 0.096 (P = 0.5227). Five minutes after irradiation, mean X-ray-induced foci (excess foci) were 0.145 ± 0.021/cell without and 0.112 ± 0.019/cell after 15 minute preincubation with radioprotective agents (P < 0.0001). Fifteen minutes after irradiation, excess foci levels were lower due to DSB repair: the mean was 0.116 ± 0.016/cell in nontreated and 0.088 ± 0.018/cell in treated cells (P < 0.0001). Preincubation with the antioxidants for 60 minutes led to a further reduction of γ-H2AX foci levels. Addition of antioxidants after irradiation did not lead to a reduction of X-ray-induced γ-H2AX foci, neither 5 (P = 0.6905) nor 15 minutes after irradiation (P = 0.8413). In the in-vivo/in-vitro experiments, pre-exposure levels ranged from 0.077 to 0.101/cell. Mean excess foci levels (± standard deviation), measured 5 minutes after 10 mGy X-ray exposure, were 0.140 ± 0.012/cell prior to radioprotectants, and 0.102 ± 0.013/cell 15 minutes, 0.078 ± 0.015/cell 30 minutes, 0.058 ± 0.012/cell 60 minutes, 0.055 ± 0.010/cell 120 minutes, 0.061 ± 0.018/cell 180 minutes, and 0.060 ± 0.018/cell 300 minutes after oral pretreatment with the antioxidant (P < 0.0001). Statistic testing showed significantly lower foci levels after all the time points between 15 and 300 minutes after pretreatment compared with the control values (P < 0.01). These experiments and results were published in *Radiology* in 2012 [47]. However, despite these promising results, future research has to prove the effect of distinct substances in randomized controlled patient studies.

Conclusions

With the help of γ-H2AX immunofluorescence microscopy it is possible to reliably estimate radiation-induced DNA DSBs in the dose range of diagnostic and interventional radiology procedures. The DSB induction correlates well with the dose delivered, but also reflects the influence of patients' individual factors (e.g. repair capacity, application of iodinated contrast agent, etc.). This latter capability of the test may be especially important in understanding further the variability, and possible genetic explanations, of responses to radiation exposure. Radiation damage depends also on individual study parameters (e.g. tube voltage), furthermore new technologies, such as "Flash-CT" may lead to a reduction in the DBS induction. Thus individual adjustment of examination protocols to the patient may be mandatory not only for image quality reasons, but also for radiation protection. Our method of detecting DNA DSBs may provide actual direct patient findings of the effect of various adjustments or interventions on the damage experienced by patients, on an individual basis. Thereby this may provide truly patient-centered medical practice. With the aid of biological phantom models it will hopefully be possible to estimate the local radiation damage in exposed tissues. A very provocative, forward-looking branch of research is the value of antioxidants and glutathione-elevating enzymes in radiation protection.

Conclusions about research in Radiology

We provided above two examples of ongoing research that are at virtually opposite ends of the research spectrum, revealing the breadth of research that is now part of the scope of modern Radiology: from purely patient psychology research to research that is founded upon exact measuring of damage to cells by medical radiation. To the present time these extremes of research have not been fully embraced by Radiology. We believe they should be in the future.

In Dostoyevsky's *The Brothers Karamazov*, one of the chapters, "The Grand Inquisitor," describes how Christ returns to 16th-century Spain and begins performing miracles. He is observed by the Grand Inquisitor to be creating a considerable stir by his miracle working. The Grand Inquisitor promptly has him imprisoned, and visits Christ late at night. Their dialogue is worth reading. In a similar fashion, we could envisage Sir Alexander Fleming returning to observe how medical research is conducted since the days when he discovered penicillin. In our opinion, in the early part of the 20th century the appreciation of the value of research by medical centers was based on the merits of the quality of the scientific work itself. Through the 1950s a shift began so that the amount of funding raised by the researcher became extremely important in the eyes of senior Health Care System administration, and by the 1970s and 1980s, the amount of money they raised for the institution became approximately of equivalent importance. By the 1990s the amount of money overtook the science itself in importance, and in the environment of the early part of the 21st century, the money has become virtually everything, and the science secondary. We espouse the return to the emphasis on the science itself as being of preeminent importance. This will be expanded in the second edition of this work; but critical aspects are the changing of culture of the NIH (so that instead of the agency advertising for grant submissions and having the voluminous grant-writing process being the barrier to entry, the quality of the science becomes the barrier), and the minimization of nepotism. It has been estimated that only 5% of NIH funding translates into useful discoveries [48, 49], and this reflects the above limitations. Actually, the so-called "valley of death" is where laboratory discoveries remain, creating the gap between bench research and clinical application [49]. Roberts et al. discuss a possible and very plausible explanation, which is the decline of the clinician scientist as the percentage of MDs receiving NIH funding has drastically decreased compared with PhDs [49]. They go further: "The growing gap between the research and clinical enterprises has resulted in fewer scientists with a true understanding of clinical problems as well as scientists who are unable to or uninterested in gleaning new basic research hypotheses from failed clinical trials" [49]. The NIH (and other major agencies) should seek out researchers who have accomplished important scientific discoveries using a task force, and offer to fund them based on the quality of their work and also on their potential to truly bring basic research into clinical usefulness [50–52]. There should be strict time limits of how long individuals are involved in the fund allocation process by granting agencies (two 4-year terms at most), and evidence of preferential-funding should be specifically prosecuted.

References

1. Hillman BJ. The past 25 years in medical imaging research: A memoir. Radiology 2000; 214:11–14.
2. Thrall JH. Building research programs in diagnostic radiology. Part I. Framing the issues. Radiology 2006; 241:646–650.
3. Virapongse C, Emerson S, Li KC, et al. Research resources in academic radiology. Radiology 1990; 175:247–251.
4. Ehman RL, Cruea RL. Academy of Radiology Research—Annual Update 2012. Available online at: http://www.acadrad.org/annualreport/AcademyAnnualUpdate 2012.pdf, [accessed on March 1, 2013].
5. Alderson PO, Bresolin LB, Becker GJ, et al. Enhancing research in academic radiology departments: Recommendations of the 2003 Consensus Conference. Radiology 2004; 232:405–408.

6. Chan S, Gunderman RB. Emerging strategic themes for guiding change in academic radiology departments. Radiology 2005; 236:430–440.

7. Thrall JH. Building research programs in diagnostic radiology. Part III. Clinical and translational research. Radiology 2007; 243:5–9.

8. Thrall JH. Building research programs in diagnostic radiology. Part II. Basic research. Radiology 2007; 242:329–333.

9. Bleyer A, Welch HG. Effect of three decades of screening mammography on breast-cancer incidence. N Engl J Med 2012; 367:1998–2005.

10. Current protocols. American College of Radiology Imaging Network 2012. Available online at: http://www.acrin.org/PROTOCOLSUMMARYTABLE.aspx. [accessed March 1, 2013].

11. Coalition for Imaging & Bioengineering Research Web site. Available online at: http://www.imagingcoalition.org/national-institutes-of-health/. [accessed on March 1, 2013].

12. PBS Frontline. Facing Ddeath: The facts and figures 2010. Available online at: http://www.pbs.org/wgbh/pages/frontline/facing-death/facts-and-figures/. [accessed on March 1, 2013].

13. Jacobs LM, Burns K, Bennett Jacobs B. Trauma death: Views of the public and trauma professionals on death and dying from injuries. Arch Surg 2008; 143:730–735.

14. Zier LS, Burack JH, Micco G, et al. Doubt and belief in physicians' ability to prognosticate during critical illness: the perspective of surrogate decision makers. Crit Care Med 2008; 36:2341–2347.

15. Balboni TA, Vanderwerker LC, Block SD, et al. Religiousness and spiritual support among advanced cancer patients and associations with end-of-life treatment preferences and quality of life. J Clin Oncol 2007; 25:555–560.

16. Phelps AC, Maciejewski PK, Nilsson M, et al. Religious coping and use of intensive life-prolonging care near death in patients with advanced cancer. JAMA 2009; 301:1140–1147.

17. True G, Phipps EJ, Braitman LE, et al. Treatment preferences and advance care planning at end of life: The role of ethnicity and spiritual coping in cancer patients. Ann Behav Med 2005; 30:174–179.

18. Maciejewski PK, Phelps AC, Kacel EL, et al. Religious coping and behavioral disengagement: Opposing influences on advance care planning and receipt of intensive care near death. Psychooncology 2012; 21:714–723.

19. Balboni TA, Paulk ME, Balboni MJ, et al. Provision of spiritual care to patients with advanced cancer: associations with medical care and quality of life near death. J Clin Oncol 2010; 28:445–452.

20. Byock I. The Best Care Possible: A Physician's Quest to Transform Care Through the End of Life. London, UK: Penguins Books Ltd, 2012.

21. Puchalski CM, Ferrell B. Making Health Care Whole: Integrating Spirituality into Patient Care. Conshohocken, PA: Templeton Press, 2010.

22. Holzel BK, Carmody J, Vangel M, et al. Mindfulness practice leads to increases in regional brain gray matter density. Psychiatry Res 2011; 191:36–43.

23. Miller JF. Hope: A construct central to nursing. Nursing Forum 2007; 42:12–19.

24. Morrison RS, Meier DE. Clinical practice. Palliative care. N Engl J Med 2004; 350:2582–2590.

25. Benzein E, Norberg A, Saveman BI. The meaning of the lived experience of hope in patients with cancer in palliative home care. Palliat Med 2001; 15:117–126.

26. Hall DE, Meador KG, Koenig HG. Measuring religiousness in health research: Review and critique. J Relig Health 2008; 47:134–163.

27. Yates P. Towards a reconceptualization of hope for patients with a diagnosis of cancer. J Adv Nurs 1993; 18:701–706.

28. Penson J. A hope is not a promise: Fostering hope within palliative care. Int J Palliat Nurs 2000; 6:94–98.

29. Snyder CR, Feldman DB, Taylor JD, et al. The roles of hopeful thinking in preventing problems and enhancing strengths. Applied & Preventive Psychology 2000; 9.

30. McGeer V. The art of good hope. The Annals of the American Academy of Political and Social Science 2004; 592:100–127.

31. Mok E, Lau KP, Lam WM, et al. Health-care professionals' perspective on hope in the palliative care setting. J Palliat Med 2010; 13:877–883.

32. Rothkamm K, Lobrich M. Evidence for a lack of DNA double-strand break repair in human cells exposed to very low x-ray doses. Proc Natl Acad Sci USA 2003; 100:5057–5062.

33. Lobrich M, Rief N, Kuhne M, et al. In vivo formation and repair of DNA double-strand breaks after computed tomography examinations. Proc Natl Acad Sci U S A 2005; 102:8984–8989.

34. Rothkamm K, Balroop S, Shekhdar J, et al. Leukocyte DNA damage after multidetector row CT: A quantitative biomarker of low-level radiation exposure. Radiology 2007; 242:244–251.

35. Schuhbaeck A, Achenbach S, Layritz C, et al. Image quality of ultra-low radiation exposure coronary CT angiography with an effective dose <0.1 mSv using high-pitch spiral acquisition and raw data-based iterative reconstruction. Eur Radiol 2013; 23:597–606.

36. Kuefner MA, Hinkmann FM, Alibek S, et al. Reduction of X-ray induced DNA double-strand breaks in blood lymphocytes during coronary CT angiography using high-pitch spiral data acquisition with prospective ECG-triggering. Invest Radiol 2010; 45:182–187.

37. Kuefner MA, Grudzenski S, Hamann J, et al. Effect of CT scan protocols on x-ray-induced DNA double-strand breaks in blood lymphocytes of patients undergoing coronary CT angiography. Eur Radiol 2010; 20:2917–2924.

38. Brand M, Sommer M, Achenbach S, et al. X-ray induced DNA double-strand breaks in coronary CT angiography: Comparison of sequential, low-pitch helical and high-pitch helical data acquisition. Eur J Radiol 2012; 81:e357–362.

39. Grudzenski S, Kuefner MA, Heckmann MB, et al. Contrast medium-enhanced radiation damage caused by CT examinations. Radiology 2009; 253:706–714.

40. Geisel D, Heverhagen JT, Kalinowski M, et al. DNA double-strand breaks after percutaneous transluminal angioplasty. Radiology 2008; 248:852–859.

41. Beels L, Bacher K, De Wolf D, et al. Gamma-H2AX foci as a biomarker for patient X-ray exposure in pediatric cardiac catheterization: are we underestimating radiation risks? Circulation 2009; 120:1903–1909.

42. Kuefner MA, Grudzenski S, Schwab SA, et al. DNA double-strand breaks and their repair in blood lymphocytes of patients undergoing angiographic procedures. Invest Radiol 2009; 44:440–446.

43. Kuefner MA, Grudzenski S, Schwab SA, et al. X-ray-induced DNA double-strand breaks after angiographic examinations of different anatomic regions. Rofo 2009; 181:374–380.

44. May MS, Brand M, Wuest W, et al. Induction and repair of DNA double-strand breaks in blood lymphocytes of patients undergoing (18)F-FDG PET/CT examinations. Eur J Nucl Med Mol Imaging 2012; 39:1712–1719.

45. Reliene R, Pollard JM, Sobol Z, et al. N-acetyl cysteine protects against ionizing radiation-induced DNA damage but not against cell killing in yeast and mammals. Mutat Res 2009; 665:37–43.

46. Weiss JF, Landauer MR. Protection against ionizing radiation by antioxidant nutrients and phytochemicals. Toxicology 2003; 189:1–20.

47. Kuefner MA, Brand M, Ehrlich J, et al. Effect of antioxidants on X-ray-induced gamma-H2AX foci in human blood lymphocytes: Preliminary observations. Radiology 2012; 264:59–67.

48. Sachs F. Is the NIH budget saturated? Why hasn't more funding meant more publications? The Scientist 2007. Available online at: http://www.the-scientist. com/?articles.view/articleNo/25416/title/Is-the-NIH-budget-saturated-/. [accessed on March 1, 2013].

49. Roberts SF, Fischhoff MA, Sakowski SA, et al. Perspective: Transforming science into medicine: How clinician-scientists can build bridges across research's "valley of death". Acad Med 2012; 87:266–270.

50. Costello LC. Perspective: Is NIH funding the "best science by the best scientists"? A critique of the NIH R01 research grant review policies. Acad Med 2010; 85:775–779.

51. Gelijns AC, Gabriel SE. Looking beyond translation—integrating clinical research with medical practice. N Engl J Med 2012; 366:1659–1661.

52. Lenfant C. Shattuck lecture—clinical research to clinical practice—lost in translation? N Engl J Med 2003; 349:868–874.

Subject index

Health Care Reform in Radiology, First Edition. Richard C. Semelka and Jorge Elias Jr.
© 2013 John Wiley & Sons, Inc. Published 2013 by John Wiley & Sons, Inc.